MENOPAUSE WITHOUT MEDICINE

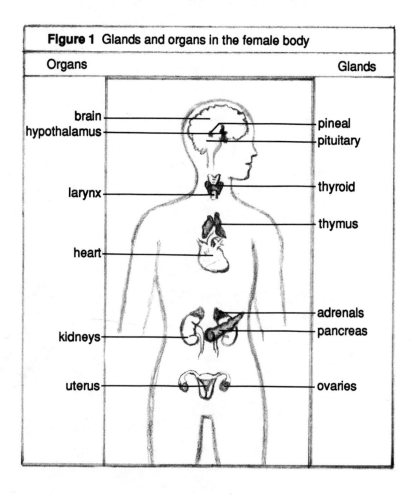

Figure 1 Glands and organs in the female body

Organs

Glands

brain

hypothalamus

larynx

heart

kidneys

uterus

pineal

pituitary

thyroid

thymus

adrenals

pancreas

ovaries

MENOPAUSE WITHOUT MEDICINE

Feel Healthy,
Look Younger,
Live Longer

LINDA OJEDA, PH.D.

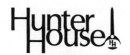

First U.S. edition published in 1989 by Hunter House

Hunter House Inc., Publishers
P.O. Box 847
Claremont, CA 91711

Library of Congress Cataloging in Publication Data:

Ojeda, Linda.
    Menopause without medicine.

    Bibliography: p. 264
    Includes index.
    1. Menopause. I. Title. [DNLM: 1. Menopause—popular works.
WP 580 039m]
RG186.0325   1989   618.1'75   87-22531
ISBN 0-89793-049-5 (cloth)
ISBN 0-89793-040-1 (paper)

Book design by Qalagraphia
Cover design by Teri Robertson
Line art and illustrations by Daniel Nyiri
Copy editing by Betty Bartelme, Lisa Kirk and Judy Selhorst
Editorial manager: Jennifer D. Trzyna
Production manager: Paul J. Frindt
Set in 11/13 Goudy by 847 Communications, Claremont, CA
Printed by Cushing-Malloy, Inc., Ann Arbor, MI
Manufactured in the United States of America

10 9 8 7 6 5 4 3 2 1

618.75
039m

082893

To my husband, Roland

Table of Contents

—————————— ❧ ——————————

Throughout the text, numbers in parentheses refer to the Notes, which are arranged by chapter and start on page 264.

Acknowledgements

— ❧ —

Many people have contributed to this book by providing me with both information and inspiration. I thank you all.

My special thanks also go—

to those who helped distribute my questionnaire when I was researching this book: Professors David Steele, Ph.D., and Chris George, Ph.D. of California Polytechnic Institute, Pomona, and exercise instructors Marilyn Grant and Pat DeBever of the Whittier YMCA;

to four very special ladies who agreed to be interviewed for this book, and who have made unique contributions to women's health: Bobbe Sommer, Ph.D., Vera Brown, Sheila Cluff, and Mary Lins;

to the British physicians who gave of their valuable time to show me their clinics and talk candidly with me about their research, opinions, and views on menopause: John Studd, MRCOG, Malcolm Whitehead, MRCOG, Nick Siddle, M.D., John Moran, M.D., and Barbara Evans, M.D.;

to the editors who cut, revised and polished so well: Elizabeth Bartelme, Lisa Kirk, and Judy Selhorst;

to a very talented illustrator, Daniel Nyiri;

to the entire staff at Hunter House, who participated in making this book a reality: Paul Frindt, Jennifer Trzyna, Lou Caughman, and especially, my publisher and friend, Kiran Rana;

and finally, to my family, my support system: Roland, Jill, and Joey.

Foreword

A virtual revolution has taken place in the field of applied clinical biochemistry over the past decade. This has come about as a result of our increased recognition of the important part that nutrition plays in health. The book you now hold in your hands, *Menopause Without Medicine*, is both a testament to and an agent of this revolution.

In the past, we considered genetic inheritance the major factor in human health. In recent years, however, we have learned much more about how various nutrients modulate human biology. While our genes dictate predispositions to specific problems, the nutritional environment and our lifestyle habits alter the genetic risk. In fact, these factors may be *more* important in determining the health patterns of midlife and later age than our genes.

As a result, I believe that understanding the basics of proper nutrition and the important role it plays in the aging process is vital for everyone.

Menopause Without Medicine is a well-researched, comprehensive health guide for women approaching or going through menopause. It offers them a program to ease the transition, as well as specific nutritional remedies for common menopausal symptoms. Dr. Ojeda addresses the crucial physical problems associated with menopause: hot flashes, vaginal dryness, and osteoporosis. She explains them in terms that are easy to understand and provides sound nutritional advice for counteracting or minimizing these conditions.

Our society, focused on youth, must grow to understand that old age is not a disease. The problems we associate with aging and menopause are *not* inevitable. Dr. Ojeda lays proper stress on the necessity of preparing the body in the early years so that later symptoms will be minimal. Because she has carefully evaluated many scientific and clinical studies, and collected in one place the best of what we currently know about nutritional relief for the symptoms of menopause, the *information* in *Menopause Without*

Medicine is valuable to all women.

Equally important is the author's *attitude*, which is that women must take care of their health on all fronts: physical, mental, and emotional. Her book goes beyond the physical aspects to discuss the effects of cultural attitudes and the emotions associated with menopause. In writing about issues like self-image and beauty care, sexuality and depression, Dr. Ojeda addresses the real concerns of women who want to deal positively with all the changes that accompany the climacteric.

Perhaps most important is Dr. Ojeda's *purpose* in writing this book: to empower women entering a new phase, to offer them hope and a greater measure of control over their lives. I believe *Menopause Without Medicine* is a book that can help most women in their quest for good health. It will certainly help *all* women to prepare for menopause with understanding, confidence, serenity and even, it is to be hoped, joyful anticipation.

Jeffrey S. Bland, Ph.D.

PART I

Menopause: Myth and Reality

Chapter 1

The Best Is Yet to Come

> The woman who wants her second chance
> years to be the best of all has to work at shap-
> ing her future.
>> —Dr. Joyce Brothers, *Better than Ever*

NEGATIVE MISCONCEPTIONS

Our society today, the society most of us have grown up in, is clearly youth-oriented. As much as we would like to believe that
vitality and beauty are possible at any age, magazines and television continue to remind us that the emphasis on young bodies
still exists. Today, partly as a result of the women's movement and
partly because of an increasing interest in health and fitness
among all ages, that tendency is changing—slowly, perhaps, but
very surely. Until recently, the image of the happy, capable, well-
groomed, and sexy mature woman was virtually nonexistent. Instead, society tended to picture her as a grandmother figure: a
pleasingly plump, matronly woman who is subdued and sexually
neutral, and whose life revolves around dentures, laxatives, digestive aids, and support hose.

Menopause has almost never been a particularly positive or
uplifting topic. Many earlier medical texts list it as a disease or an

unnatural phenomenon. The terms most commonly used to describe it are *climacteric, endocrine starvation, involutionary years, female trouble*, and a *living decay*. No wonder women tend to dread the so-called change of life. Descriptions such as these can significantly affect a woman's attitudes and emotional responses to menopause, especially if she is poorly informed. Many physical and psychological reactions to menopause may be directly related to this long-term negative conditioning.

Robert Wilson, in his supposedly pro-female book *Feminine Forever*, titles one of his chapters "The Loss of Womanhood and the Loss of Good Health."(1) He describes the menopausal woman as becoming the equivalent of a eunuch—unbearable, suicidal, incapacitated, and incapable of rationally perceiving her own situation. Equally degrading to women is the work of Dr. David Reuben, author of the popular book *Everything You Always Wanted to Know About Sex*. This male authority maintains that the essence of femininity is tied to a woman's ovaries; therefore, once the estrogen is virtually shut off, a woman comes as close as she can to being a man. Such a woman is not really a man, he explains, but she is no longer a functional woman; according to Reuben, menopausal women live in the "world of intersex."(2) This is absurd. A woman's femininity is not defined by the amount of estrogen in her body any more than a man's masculinity is measured by his testosterone output.

For some people, the idea of physical menopause, the cessation of the menstrual cycle and the end of fertility, brings to mind the image of an emotionally distraught, sometimes hysterical woman unable to cope with daily life, a woman somehow drained of her sexuality and her usefulness, who typically screams at her family, cries frequently, and cannot make the simplest decision. *This is myth.* The reality is that women in menopause are facing what can be the best years of their lives.

The thought of menopause should not and need not produce anxiety. A study of other societies shows that the stereotype of the irrational woman is not universal, that our negative reactions to common physiological processes, such as menstruation and menopause, are culturally engendered. In countries where age is venerated and elders enjoy respect for their experience and wisdom, older women seem to manifest fewer physical and psychological symptoms. For example, South African, Asian, and Arabic women, who, it is said, welcome the end of the childbearing years, are reported to have positive attitudes about the change of life. Where there are different predefined concepts, aging seems to be more natural, less confused, and not overlaid with negative images.(3)

The fact is that menopause, like menarche, is inevitable and totally natural. It is *another* change of life, not *the* change, and life is but a series of changes. We grow older not only after a certain age, but after birth itself. How smoothly a woman adapts to any change in her life depends largely on the health of her total being—her body, her mind, and her spirit.

It is imperative that women understand the workings of their bodies, with all the various hormonal fluctuations, in order to avoid unnecessary fear, anxiety, and stress. Understanding can also enhance a woman's experience of her changing body. It is time to shed the myths and misconceptions about menopause that our society has harbored and instead build a foundation for the sense of well-being that each woman deserves.

PRESENT-DAY ATTITUDES

I was raised in an era when normal female topics, such as menstruation and menopause, were not openly discussed even among close friends. Our bodies, we were led to believe, were too mysterious to understand and too base to mention. Our intimate parts were ignored as if they did not exist. Even today, unfortunately, our childhood attitudes prevent many of us from learning, accepting, and openly discussing our bodies, our problems, and our feelings about them.

As I was gathering data for this book, I wondered how thinking had changed from my early experiences. Had women younger than me been subject to the same inhibitions concerning their sexuality, or had they become more enlightened?

I decided to conduct my own survey of women's attitudes about menopause, the so-called change of life. Researchers and books had given me a good idea about it; however, the idea of accumulating firsthand accounts had a special appeal.

This survey included several questions, some based on the much larger questionnaire of the Boston Women's Health Collective, and others I just wanted to ask. Mine was a small, informal study of 100 women; I consider it in no way to be scientific. The respondents, all from Southern California, included students at California State Polytechnic University, Pomona, and middle-class homemakers and working mothers enrolled in the Whittier YMCA dance and exercise classes. These women can hardly be considered a wide cross-section of society, yet I feel that their responses indicate current trends in attitudes toward menopause. The Boston survey, which was conducted ten years ago by the collective authors of *Our Bodies, Ourselves*, even though considerably larger (2,000 women), was likewise less than scientific, because it, too, was given to a select group of women rather than to a random sample.

The primary question— "What do you think about when you hear the word menopause?"—was similar to that of the Boston study. Generally, my smaller survey corroborated the findings of the larger group. About half the women shared positive feelings or gave descriptive, neutral responses. Typical answers included "It's part of a woman's cycle"; "a normal, happy experience"; "finally, the end of monthly periods"; "a physiological process that all women go through in their midyears"; "no problem." The other half were less accepting of the idea: "It indicates old age and the end of youth"; "a very depressing and difficult time to deal with"; "I'm not looking forward to it"; "a traumatic experience in a woman's life, where emotions run rampant for a few years, then everything falls back into place"; "a very unpleasant time in a woman's life"; "a time of depression, frustration, and hot flashes."

There are a few interesting discrepancies between my survey and the larger Boston survey. The Boston survey found that younger women were generally more anxious and negative about menopause, whereas older women were more matter-of-fact.(4) The authors suggest that this might indicate that younger women tend to have a somewhat distorted view of the menopausal experience. Moreover, they speculate that possibly the older women in their sample represent a unique group of fairly active women (two-thirds of them had jobs outside the home during and/or after menopause) who generally had positive self-images.

In my survey, the proportions of older and younger women with positive attitudes are about even. The younger women in my survey may have answered differently because, having been drawn primarily from a college sex education class, they were relatively well informed about the physiological process of menopause. If they had been fearful or negative before taking the class, their outlooks probably changed by the end of the quarter. This makes a strong case for providing knowledge to help reduce fear and anxiety.

On my survey, one question was, "Do you remember what your mother, aunt, or friend experienced when she went through menopause?" Very few respondents remembered their mothers or other relatives experiencing the change, or even discussing the subject at all. This did not surprise me. As I mentioned before, when I was growing up, any topic remotely related to sex was closely guarded, if discussed at all. If women agonized over menopause, they usually suffered in silence.

The possibility of gaining weight concerned almost everyone in my sample. Surprisingly, many did not accept that weight gain was inevitable. Many women, especially those who exercised regularly, felt that whether or not they gained extra pounds during menopause was a matter of self-control. By not accepting fate as an excuse for putting on weight at menopause, these women will most likely make the adjustments necessary to maintain their premenopausal figures.

Appearance in general did not seem to concern the majority of respondents as did weight gain. The consensus was that wrinkles, hair color and texture, age spots, and so on are genetically determined and unavoidable. Something could always be done to minimize the signs of aging using cosmetic surgery, makeup, and beauty aids. Some women were not uncomfortable about wrinkles and such, and for them, such age-related changes were not a significant issue. In any case, I was glad to find that the majority of women did not feel they would be "less of a woman" after menopause.

Slightly more than half of my respondents stated unequivocally that they would not under any circumstances take hormones. The remainder were divided between maybe and yes, if the doctor prescribes them. Only a few left the decision entirely to the physician. The need for hormone therapy has to be evaluated on an individual basis. I would only suggest that women themselves be fully informed about the risks and benefits before deciding one way or another. Ultimately, the decision should be a woman's own, based on her research, her doctor's recommendation, and a large measure of her own common sense.

THE SECOND CHANCE YEARS

Women in menopause are facing what can be the best years of their lives. The life span of the modern woman is currently 78 years, and gerontologists anticipate that it will soon increase to 80. Even the conservative American Medical Association's Council on Medical Services boldly asserts that with intelligent living we could all live to be 90 or 100 years old. This means that, before too many more decades have passed, the average woman may be living as many years after menopause as she lived before it. We need to be concerned with enhancing the quality of those years. Just think—if a woman has devoted the first half or third of her life to raising a family, she can still have time to go back to college, start a new career, travel, write the great American novel, learn French, or climb Mount Everest. We don't have to restrict our goals to one career or one life path. Our options increase, especially when we are mentally and physically prepared to exercise them.

We must not underestimate the emotional impact that menopause has on many women. Psychologist Helene Deutsch calls the psychological experience of menopause the most trying time of a woman's life, and Juanita Williams agrees: "Although it is the manifest sign of the end of reproductive life, its symbolic meanings invest it with an importance which extends far beyond its biological definition."(5)

We all need to examine our cultural associations and belief systems concerning menopause. Are they based on fact or fallacy? Listed below are my responses to the most common misconceptions about menopause. What are your feelings about them?

* Menopause is not the beginning of the end.
* You will not age faster after menopause.
* You do not have to gain weight, become depressed, or lose your looks because of menopause.
* Fertility does not equal femininity.
* You do not lose interest in sex because of decreasing estrogen.
* Taking estrogen will not keep you young forever.
* Your feelings are just as genuine at menopause as at any other time of your life.
* Menopause is not mysterious; it can be understood.
* There are natural remedies to nearly all menopausal symptoms.
* It is possible to alleviate physiological and psychological symptoms of menopause by preparing physically and mentally.
* You do not have to suffer in silence; in fact, you do not have to suffer at all.

PERSONALITY TYPES AND MENOPAUSAL REACTIONS

It appears to be the case that women with certain types of personalities tend to develop certain menopausal symptoms. Although the evidence is not conclusive, I feel there is value in relaying this information, because it may apply to and help a large number of women.

Researchers have found that certain personality types find it more traumatic to adjust to changes during the menopausal years. Gynecologist Sheldon Cherry finds that women with a history of continued emotional problems have the hardest time. These include women with chronic sexual difficulties, immature women with narcissistic tendencies, women whose erotic attractiveness was the chief element of their personal worth, childless women facing the undeniable loss of fertility, and married women who feel that their meaningful years are over.(6)

Several authorities have observed that how women react emotionally to the change usually reflects how they perceive themselves as women. Particularly vulnerable, according to British physician Dr. Barbara Evans, are the women who over the years have defined their femininity in terms of bodily functions—menstruation, pregnancy, and motherhood.(7) For them, menopause represents the termination of their womanly identity; it removes the purpose of their existence. In some respects, this may be compared to the shock some men have been known to experience when forced to retire from work.

Then there is the group of women who represent another all-too-common phenomenon: women who submerge their own desires, talents, and personal growth to live totally through their children's activities and accomplishments. It is no wonder that, when their children leave home, these women undergo an emotional trauma similar to experiencing the death of a loved one. They have lost the chief component of their identity as women and as a contributing member of society. The "empty-nest syndrome" is the name given to this scenario, and it often results in depression. The midlife woman must search for a new identity in her relationship to her grown children.

The degree to which a woman accepts or fears growing older also affects the transition. The reality of getting older must be dealt with at some time in our lives. Often this time coincides with or develops with menopause. If the thought of aging, coupled with diminishing attractiveness and usefulness, frightens you, I would like to recommend a book I find particularly inspiring. In *Always a Woman*, Kaylan Pickford emphasizes the beauty to be found in all phases of life. No one part is better or to be compared to another, she tells us; each is uniquely different and special. In her own words, "While there can be beauty in life that is in the process of becoming (as in a flower bud), there is also beauty in life that has achieved itself (as in the flower in full bloom)."(8)

Research indicates that women who accept menopause as a natural condition of life are likely to breeze through it unscathed. For them, the transition is comparatively uncomplicated, uneventful, and relatively symptomless. In addition, women whose educational skills make more options available to them are reported to handle the change with relative ease.(9) Numerous studies indicate that women with professional interests, intellectual and creative outlets, and challenging responsibilities have an easier time during menopause. It is not clear exactly why active women appear to suffer less physical and emotional pain than their homebound sisters, but theories are that they have less time to dwell on their symptoms, are generally more knowledgeable about the physiological details of menopause and about their own bodies, and as a rule have higher self-esteem. Whether a particular woman's symptoms during menopause will be closely related to her personality type or feelings about herself cannot be predicted with certainty. Body chemistry is just not that simple. To portray a complex psychophysiological process such as menopause in black-and-white terms would be misleading. Each woman has a highly individual chemical makeup, genetic predisposition, and hormonal balance. Even the most secure, well-adjusted, and happy woman may have emotional symptoms during menopause. No one can predict how individual women will respond.

CREATING A POSITIVE IMAGE

What we think and believe not only determines our daily decisions, it also establishes the entire direction of our life. Attitudes shape our future, write Napoleon Hill and W. Clement Stone, authors of the best-selling book *Success Through a Positive Mental Attitude*. This is a universal law. We translate into physical reality the thoughts and attitudes we hold in our minds, no matter what they are.(10)

Our attitudes toward menopause may have been engendered by our culture and our families, but they are not unchangeable. If our ideas are counterproductive, we can choose to acknowledge the fears and anxieties we harbor and alter them. We can begin then to reverse the obstacles in our lives.

Of course, this is never as easy as it sounds. Whether you are 50 years old or 20, take stock of your belief system and your general attitudes. If you feel you are valued only for your children's or husband's accomplishments, few will acknowledge the real you. If you think that to be beautiful you must be young, your mature years will have little joy. If you are convinced that the quality of your life will vanish at 50 or 60 or 70, then it will. If you believe your health, looks, body, and mind all begin to deteriorate with the onset of menopause, they probably will.

We women are often experts at suppressing our innermost thoughts. We have learned through years of conditioning to "put on a happy face," to keep up appearances and to insist that everything is fine when our bodies and souls silently scream just the opposite.

We try so hard to please our children, parents, friends, and neighbors, to be all they would like us to be, that we lose sight of who we are and what we believe. We try to become everything to everyone, yet end up being nothing to ourselves. We carry around vestiges of ancient traditions, obsolete fears, and borrowed beliefs, promising that some day when life is less hectic we will sort everything out; and we lose touch with our true inner selves.

Many writers on menopause and the midlife phase have said that this is the perfect time to rediscover oneself, to establish new goals, to reassess values. In my opinion, the hormone changes are quite enough to deal with, and identity questions can just take a backseat. In any case, we should continually be examining the truth of our lives, not just when we reach momentous physiological transitions.

In the following chapters, I will discuss aspects of menopause and aging, as well as understanding and taking charge of our bodies; the first step is taking charge of our lives. I will tell you how to prepare, how to cope, even how to eliminate many problems and how to make the most of what nature has already given you. The rest should be much easier after that.

Chapter 2

———— ❧ ————

The Physical Reality

> We have lived through the era when happiness was a warm puppy, and the era when happiness was a dry martini, and now we have come to the era when happiness is "knowing what your uterus looks like."
>
> —Nora Ephron

DEFINING TERMS

Menopause is often confused with climacteric. However, there is a clear-cut distinction between the two, a distinction of time span. According to Edmund Novak's *Textbook of Gynecology*, menopause is the counterpart of menarche, the onset of menstrual periods, while the climacteric is the counterpart of puberty.

The word *menopause* is derived from two Greek roots: *mens*, meaning monthly, and *pause*, meaning to stop. It refers specifically to the cessation of menstruation and the termination of fertility, two events that may not necessarily happen at the same time. The process of menopause may take from one to seven years.

Climacteric, also a word of Greek origin, translates literally as "rung of the ladder." (I will leave the significance of this metaphor to you.) It is a transitional phase that lasts fifteen to twenty years,

during which ovarian function and hormone production decline
and the body readapts, and can commence any time between 40
and 60 years of age. Menopause, then is but one chapter in the saga
of the climacteric.

Menopause Compared to Climacteric

Menopause	Climacteric
* counterpart of menarche	* counterpart of puberty
* one biological event	* series of chemical changes
* cessation of periods	* transition when ovarian
* termination of fertility	function and hormones
	decline
* 1–7 years	* 15–20 years
* between ages 48–52	* between ages 40–60

WHEN WILL IT BEGIN?

For most American women today, the termination of fertility
usually takes place between 45 and 55 years of age, while most
women stop menstruating between ages 50 and 52. Interestingly,
the mean age of menopause has increased by approximately 4 years
over the past century, and gynecologists report that many women
are still menstruating well into their sixth decade.(1) Improved
nutrition, healthier life-styles, and modern medical advances are
the most notable reasons for this increase in childbearing years. To
women who have postponed having children, this news may be
encouraging.

Several studies have examined the effect of life-style on the
onset of menopause. Nutrition, in particular, appears to be a significant factor in determining when a woman enters the change of
life. A very extensive survey conducted in New Guinea found that
undernourished women start menopause around the age of 43,
while those considered more adequately nourished do not begin
until age 47.(2) Research on large population groups indicates that
European women, who supposedly engage in healthier habits than
Americans, tend toward a later menopause.

However, a wide range of additional factors influence whether menopause will arrive early or late. For instance, heredity must always be taken into account. There is some indication that women tend to follow in their mothers' footsteps: if the mother had a late menopause, it is very likely that the daughter's will be late as well. But is this nature or nurture? A growing number of scientists believe that daughters mimic their mothers, that is, they believe the influence is cultural rather than genetic. Children tend to imitate their parents' habits. Thus, how much they exercise, if they are overweight, the manner in which they handle stress, and if they smoke cigarettes or drink alcohol often depend on what their parents did. These environmental factors or role models may be at least as important as inherited tendencies.

The data from two large, independent studies involving several different countries have confirmed that smokers as a group experience earlier menopause. There are two probable explanations for this: first, nicotine, which acts on the central nervous system, may decrease the secretion of hormones, resulting in early menopause; second, nicotine may activate liver-metabolizing enzymes that alter the metabolism of the sex-related hormones.(3)

A traumatic experience may cause or appear to cause premature menopause. Prolonged stress or a crisis can cause a temporary hiatus in the production of certain hormones, and the end result may be similar to menopause. The ovaries, responding to the lack of these hormones, cease production of eggs, and subsequently of estrogen and progesterone. Periods stop and typical menopausal symptoms appear. This is known as traumatic menopause, and should not be confused with psychogenic amenorrhea, which is a temporary stopping of periods caused by tension, fatigue, exercise, low body weight, or malnutrition. If an underweight woman stops menstruating because of lack of adequate body fat, she will resume her normal cycle shortly after her weight returns to normal. In other words, psychogenic amenorrhea is a temporary problem; this is not generally the case for women going through premature or traumatic menopause.

When a woman's ovaries are irreparably damaged or when she has them surgically removed (ovariectomy or oophorectomy), she will begin menopause immediately. However, this operation should not be confused with a hysterectomy, the removal of the uterus alone. Many women are under the impression that if a woman has a hysterectomy, the change is imminent. This is not true, even though the woman will no longer be capable of having periods or becoming pregnant. If the ovaries are left intact—even if only one remains—eggs and female hormones will continue to be produced. Even if a small piece of the gland remains, it will continue to produce female hormones until menopause occurs.(4)

A hysterectomy *can*, however, cause an early menopause, perhaps even by a number of years.(5) This is possible anytime the blood circulation is cut off or compromised in any sense. Other situations involving impaired blood flow that are likely to result in an early transition include sterilization by tubal ligation, damage due to radiation treatment, chemotherapy, and certain diseases.

I would like to digress for a moment. There is considerable controversy today about unnecessary hysterectomy or ovariectomy. Because women have frequently accepted medical recommendations without asking questions or seeking second opinions, they have often been victims of unnecessary surgery. Estimates range from 15 percent to 60 percent of all such operations, depending on the study you're reading. It has been projected that within the next several years, gynecological surgeons will have removed over one-half of the uteruses in the United States. Will all these operations be performed for valid reasons? Many concerned health advocates think not.

The decision to have one's female organs removed is a serious matter. Several books offer guidelines on when hysterectomies may be indicated, and when they are normally performed but are not compulsory. For an excellent discussion of this subject, I recommend *The New Our Bodies, Ourselves*, by the Boston Women's Health Book Collective. If you are faced with this question, begin by gathering as much information as you can, both pro and con. Ask your physician why surgery is indicated, what exactly is to be removed, what your alternatives are, and what the future implications are. Do not be embarrassed or afraid to ask these questions—it is *your* body. Once you are clear about the basis for the diagnosis, get a second opinion. Make sure before you go ahead that you are satisfied this is the right choice for you. If surgery is unavoidable (and it may be your *only* option), then prepare emotionally and nutritionally to minimize any aftereffects. A healthy mind and a strong body are the best guarantees of a smooth operation and a quick recovery.

Now, let's return to the factors that affect the onset of menopause. As discussed, when estrogen is diminished in any way, menopause is likely to begin early. The biological clock may also operate in reverse: should the premenopausal supply of estrogen continue as usual, the process will be delayed.

One common condition that can delay menopause is an excess of body fat. Overweight women menstruate longer than their thinner sisters because their bodies manufacture greater amounts of estrogen. Estrogen is not produced only in the ovaries, but also in the fatty tissues of the body from another hormone, androstenedione. Thus, the more fat a woman carries, the more estrogen she creates. I suppose this could be construed as one "natural" way to postpone menopause, but it is certainly not the wisest. For one thing, an overabundance of circulating estrogen greatly increases the risk of estrogen-based cancers.

Certain diseases have also been known to provoke the endocrine system into extending estrogen production. Although the evidence is not conclusive, physicians have observed that women with cancer of the breast and uterus, women who have fibroids, and women who are diabetic may expect menopause to come somewhat later than the average age.

Factors that May Influence the Timing of the Onset of Menopause

Earlier	Later
genetics	
stress	
drugs	
underweight	overweight
hysterectomy	cancer of breast or uterus
tubal ligation	fibroids
damaged female organs	diabetes
smoking	
malnutrition	

WHO EXPERIENCES SYMPTOMS?

It has been estimated that 75–80 percent of women passing through menopause experience one or more symptoms, but only 10–35 percent are affected strongly enough to seek professional help. While it is impossible to predict who will or will not suffer severe symptoms, certain generalizations can be made.(6)

Characteristics of Women
Likely to Pass through Menopause Undisturbed

* relatively late onset of menstruation
* never been married
* never been pregnant
* gave birth after age 40
* relatively high income
* better educated

Characteristics of Women
Likely to Suffer Severe Menopausal Symptoms

* premenstrual syndrome sufferer
* had premature menopause
* had artificial menopause (oophorectomy)

It is obvious from the above lists that physiology is only one piece of the menopausal puzzle—and probably the easiest part to understand. It is easy to understand why women are bothered by symptoms after a hysterectomy, but why should women who have never been married or women who have had a child after age 40 be less likely to experience these symptoms? Is there another underlying common denominator—life-style, education, diet—that might explain these parallels? Future research must address these questions.

Generally, the *rate* at which estrogen levels drop seems to influence the number and severity of menopausal symptoms. Usually, these follow one of three patterns, explained below.

* *Pattern A: abrupt ending.* This is the immediate cessation of menstrual periods, where periods stop
  without any prior warning. It is fairly uncommon,
  since, in most cases, the ovaries stop functioning
  gradually. If the estrogen supply stops suddenly, the
  chances of a woman's experiencing symptoms are
  greater. However, not all women follow the norm.
  Menopause researcher Rosetta Reitz found a group
  whose periods stopped abruptly, yet who complained
  of relatively few symptoms.(7) She presumed these
  women had a high threshold for discomfort. This
  suggests that, while there are definable patterns, it is
  difficult to predict how any one woman will go
  through the change.

* *Pattern B: gradual ending.* This is a more common occurrence, involving a progressive decline in both the
  amount and duration of the menstrual flow. Typically, periods become shorter, delayed, or skipped; finally, they terminate altogether. A woman may not
  even be aware of the irregularity of her cycles. More
  important, if the ovaries atrophy slowly, if the organs
  they stimulate are not hypersensitive, and they continue to supply a sustaining amount of estrogen,
  symptoms are insignificant.(8)

* *Pattern C: irregular ending.* Irregular menstrual patterns are also relatively common. The flow may be
  sporadic; it may become heavier, lighter, or alternate
  monthly. The number of days between periods may
  increase or decrease. Some women may go an entire
  year without one period, and then, without warning,
  start menstruating again. Many "change-of-life
  babies" have been born because women thought
  they were "safe." Doctors now urge women to continue birth control for two years after their last
  menstrual period.

Numerous researchers, searching for possible relationships
among roles, behavior, and a tendency toward menopausal dis-

tress, have found that there is clearly a psychological component involved in menopausal distress.(9) How much of a woman's discomfort is physical and how much is a response to cultural expectations and her own belief system is difficult to determine. Each woman's symptoms and physical reactions may be totally genuine and yet nothing like those of her friends.

THE MENSTRUAL CYCLE EXPLAINED

To have a good understanding of the ways in which a woman's body changes from age 40 to age 60, it helps to have a clear understanding of the menstrual cycle. Even in this age of health consciousness and fitness, too many women do not know what is occurring monthly in their bodies. Understanding how your body works is critical to taking charge of your health and your life. Even if you believe you understand the process of menstruation, please don't gloss over this section; read it carefully—you may increase your body awareness.

The female menstrual cycle is the entire 28- or 29-day period that repeats itself monthly for a woman's fertile life. It involves an interplay among the brain, the ovaries, and four primary hormones, two secreted at each location (see Figure 2). The release of these hormones primarily stimulates the cells lining the uterus in preparation for a possible pregnancy. The uterine lining, or endometrium, is built up in the first part of the cycle and shed during the menstrual period.

A cycle characteristically has no beginning or end, but for the purpose of explanation, we start the physical stages of the menstrual cycle at the hypothalamus, an endocrine gland in the brain. Commonly referred to as the master controller, the hypothalamus plays a key role in many basic bodily functions such as body temperature, water balance, metabolic rate, appetite regulation, sleep patterns, and tolerance to stress. The hypothalamus sends a message in the form of a hormone to the anterior pituitary gland, another endocrine gland located just below it. The tiny pituitary responds to the message by secreting the first hormone of the cycle, called follicle-stimulating hormone (FSH). Like all endocrine hormones, FSH is a messenger travel-

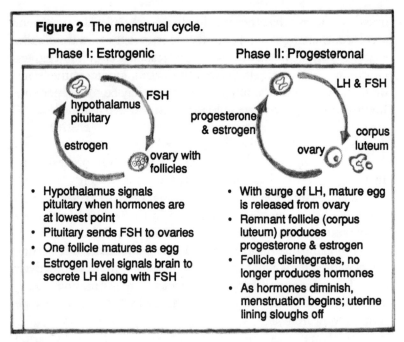

Figure 2 The menstrual cycle.

Phase I: Estrogenic   Phase II: Progesteronal

FSH — hypothalamus pituitary — estrogen — ovary with follicles

LH & FSH — progesterone & estrogen — corpus luteum — ovary

- Hypothalamus signals pituitary when hormones are at lowest point
- Pituitary sends FSH to ovaries
- One follicle matures as egg
- Estrogen level signals brain to secrete LH along with FSH

- With surge of LH, mature egg is released from ovary
- Remnant follicle (corpus luteum) produces progesterone & estrogen
- Follicle disintegrates, no longer produces hormones
- As hormones diminish, menstruation begins; uterine lining sloughs off

ing from one organ to act on another part of the body, in this case, the ovaries. Within the ovaries are small sacs or follicles that contain eggs and the female hormone estrogen. Stimulation from FSH causes one of the follicles to grow and, as it does, estrogen is released. When a specific amount of estrogen is circulating in the bloodstream, the pituitary, again under instructions from the hypothalamus, secretes its second hormone, luteinizing hormone (LH). By this time, the egg within the follicle is mature and ready to burst from the sac. The egg is expelled into the fallopian tubes and makes its way up into the uterus. The actual release of the egg is called *ovulation*, and it marks roughly the halfway point in the cycle. Remaining behind in the ovary, the remnant follicle is now a functioning endocrine gland, and has been renamed the *corpus luteum*. It is the corpus luteum that produces both estrogen and progesterone, the second female hormone, which is dominant in the second half of the cycle. The varying levels of the four hormones active in a typical menstrual cycle are shown in Figure 3.

If the egg is fertilized by a male sperm, it implants or attaches to the lining of the uterus and a special hormone called *chorionic gonadotrophin* is secreted. This hormone stimulates the continued secretion of estrogen and progesterone so that the now developing embryo will be nourished. Without fertilization of the egg and continued hormonal production, the corpus luteum shrivels and dies, and estrogen and progesterone secretion drops. When both hormones reach their lowest point, the thickened uterine lining is sloughed off through the vaginal opening and menstrual flow begins. Low blood levels of estrogen and progesterone act as a signal to the brain to produce FSH, and the whole process starts again.

During the cycle, it is the primary function of estrogen to increase the blood supply and thus the thickness of the endometrium in preparation for a suitable environment for fertilization, implantation, and nutrition of the early embryo. Progesterone further prepares the uterus for reception and development of the fertilized ovum by making available an adequate supply of nutrients.

THE CHANGING CYCLE

The first indication of approaching menopause is the beginning of anovulatory cycles, that is, cycles in which ovulation does not take place. Ovarian function actually begins to decline several years prior to menopause. The follicles that inhabit the ovaries gradually diminish in number from birth, reducing the initial 250,000 potential eggs to approximately 50 by age 40 and eventually none after menopause. With fewer follicles, some months may pass when menstruation does not occur. No follicle means no egg, no estrogen, no corpus luteum, no progesterone, and no period (see Figure 4). As the ovaries continue to reduce their production of estrogen and progesterone, the pituitary gland, in a desperate effort to stimulate the recalcitrant ovaries, pumps even greater amounts of FSH and LH into the blood. FSH escalates, reaching levels thirteen times that of normal cycles, while LH levels rise approximately threefold.(10) As it was explained to me by gynecologist Larry Francis, this elevation of hormones is most commonly and most easily used by physicians to test for the onset of menopause.

In the premenopausal period, the levels of the brain hor-

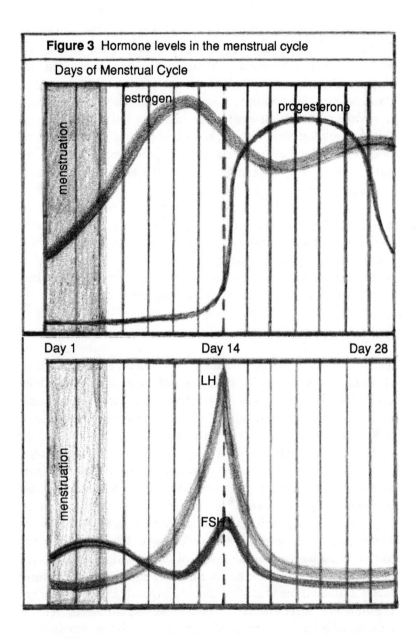

Figure 3 Hormone levels in the menstrual cycle

mones increase while the ovarian hormone levels decrease. When the ovaries stop producing eggs, progesterone, which depends on a corpus luteum for production, is no longer secreted at all. Estrogen, however, can still be manufactured by the ovaries (although in smaller amounts), by the adrenal glands, and by extraglandular sources (including, as mentioned before, certain fat cells). During the premenopausal stage, therefore, the uterine lining is being stimulated exclusively by estrogen. With no periodic shedding of the uterine lining, the tissues continue to proliferate until the lining outgrows its blood-vessel supply. It may be several months before this happens, thus, periods are often missed or irregular. When it does break down and disintegrate, it often comes off haphazardly, in uneven patches, resulting in a heavier than normal period.

Ultimately, the ovarian follicles no longer respond to the prodding of FSH and LH. Estrogen levels drop too low to cause growth in the uterine lining, menstruation ceases completely, and menopause begins. Although the mature ovary no longer ovulates, it has not ceased functioning altogether. In fact, the central region of the ovary is very actively engaged in producing hormones that are converted into estrone, the form of estrogen that remains circulating in the blood after menopause. Tests have shown that some women still show significant evidence of estrogenic activity more than twenty years after their last period.(11) Usually, the adrenal glands become the major source of postmenopausal estrogen. In fact, maintaining healthy adrenals may be one of the best ways to ensure continued estrogen production and a smoother transition.

Estrone is also converted in the body fat from another hormone, androstenedione. As was mentioned earlier, women with ample fat on their bodies not only experience menopause later because of higher estrogen levels, they also appear to suffer less discomfort than their thinner sisters. The conversion of androstenedione into estrone recently has been found to occur in the muscle, liver, kidney, brain, and possibly other unknown extraglandular sources.(12) Clearly, as the ovaries slow down, the production of estrogen diminishes, but the body readjusts, substituting other estrogen sources.

Figure 4   Pre-menopausal menstrual cycles

Phase I

Phase II

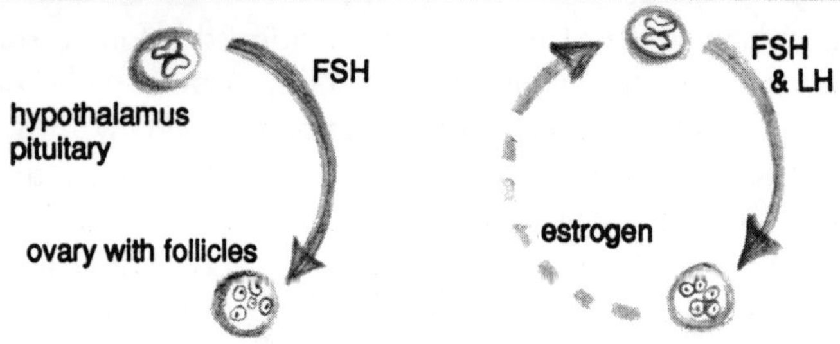

FSH

hypothalamus
pituitary

FSH
& LH

ovary with follicles

estrogen

- Hypothalamus signals
  pituitary when hormones are
  low
- Pituitary sends FSH to ovaries
- Follicle does not respond

- Follicle may not grow
  sufficiently to produce egg
- No progesterone produced;
  estrogen continues
- No period

Phase I

Phase II

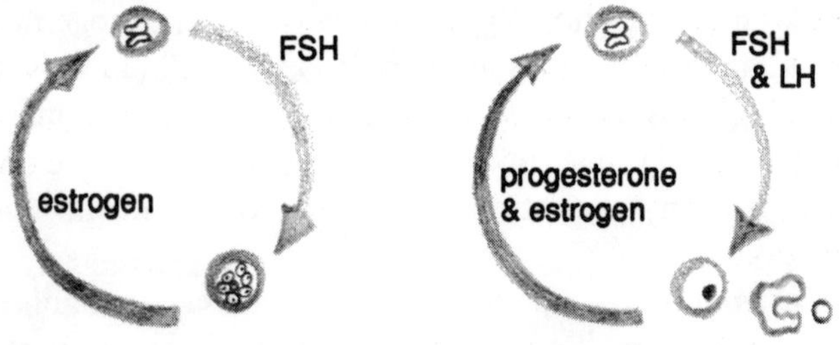

FSH

estrogen

FSH
& LH

progesterone
& estrogen

- Estrogen & progesterone still
  low
- hypothalamus signals pituitary
  to send more FSH
- Follicle may or may not
  respond
- If it does, estrogen is released

- Follicle may eventually
  produce egg
- Estrogen & progesterone
  released
- Periods erratic

What Happens to the Hormones at Menopause

* Ovarian activity decreases.
    * Estrogen is produced in decreased amounts.
    * Progesterone is no longer secreted.
* Brain hormones temporarily increase.
    * FSH and LH are produced in greater amounts.
* Estrone is produced from various sources:
    * adrenal glands,
    * body fat,
    * extraglandular sources, and
    * ovaries.

PHYSIOLOGICAL CHANGES FOLLOWING MENOPAUSE

Estrogen is of primary importance in the female life cycle. The amount of this hormone circulating in the body, the ratio of estrogen to other hormones, and its rate of change and decline prior to menopause all have effects on physical health and emotional outlook. Estrogen acts directly on the uterus, and influences other organs and tissues such as the vulva, vagina, breasts, bones, hair, skin, heart, and central nervous system. Therefore, as the level of estrogen decreases, substantial changes occur in the appearance and function of all these organs. This is not to say that every menopausal symptom is related to declining hormones— some are the natural results of aging. For example, hot flashes, the loss of vaginal lubrication, and thinning of the tissues probably are hormonally dependent, while the loss of elasticity, middle-age spread, and sagging skin most likely are not.

Most postmenopausal women will experience varying degrees of atrophic (shrinking and thinning) changes of the vagina, cervix, uterus, and ovaries. Specifically, one can expect a decrease in the size of the cervix and uterus, accompanied by a reduction in cervical mucus. Some women become more prone to bacterial infections because of the decline in cervical secretions. The *labia majora* (larger skin folds of the vagina) become thinner, flatter, paler, and less elastic. The vaginal wall shortens and loses its muscle tone as well as some of its normal secretions, sometimes making intercourse uncomfortable or painful.

Structures around the reproductive organs suffer loss of muscle tone as a result of natural aging and lack of exercise. In the extreme state, the relaxed structures fall into other organs. For example, the uterus may fall, causing the cervix to rest on or even enter the vaginal wall. A sensation of heaviness in the vaginal area or the feeling that tissue is protruding outward may indicate a descending bladder, uterus, or rectum. Lack of muscle tone may also cause the urinary sphincter muscles not to contract satisfactorily, so that urine escapes when the individual laughs, sneezes, coughs, or lifts heavy objects. Uncontrollable urinary leaking (incontinence) can be prevented and/or relieved through special exercises called "Kegel exercises," described in Chapter 8. (All of the internal muscles, in fact, can be toned and maintained through exercises that are explained in Chapter 17.)

Fat disappears from the breast tissue, reducing breasts' size, shape, and firmness. Nipples tend to become smaller and less erect. Some women report decreased sexual stimulation from the breast, but whether this is physical or psychological is undetermined. On the positive side, women who have been tormented by fibrocystic breast disease (lumpy, painful breasts) will be relieved to know that this discomfort usually subsides during or after menopause.

Aging also involves obvious changes in the hair and skin. Body hair may thin out in some women and increase in others. New growth on the upper lip and chin is ascribed to the reversed ratio of estrogen to androgen. While women always have this "male" hormone in their systems, it is only after menopause that it is physically discernible. This is because the level of estrogen has decreased, making the ratio of androgen to estrogen greater.

Wrinkling and loss of skin tone are particularly noticeable around the face, neck, and hands. Characteristic purse-string wrinkles form around the mouth and "crows' feet" develop at the corners of the eyes. Many natural preventive measures can minimize at least some fine aging lines.

There is a pervasive belief that women who take estrogen therapy or use estrogen creams appear younger; this is debatable. In an informal survey, Barbara Seaman and Gideon Seaman,

M.D., observed that estrogen users did not look more youthful; they only thought they did. On the other hand, women who did not rely on hormone therapy but were very conscientious about diet and exercise were (in the Seamans' opinion) deceptively young in appearance.(13) These well-respected researchers concluded that estrogen therapy may give women a false sense of security and prevent them from engaging in commonsense approaches to aging.

For many years, women passively accepted the "matronly" image of aging; as one gets older, body configuration alters, fat redistributes, the metabolism slows down, and there is a tendency to gain weight. Now that appears to be changing. With a little conscious effort, regular exercise, and a few less calories, women are fighting the battle of the bulge, working to maintain healthy, trim, and toned figures throughout their lives.

When estrogen levels fall, the bones suffer. Reduced estrogen activity has been directly related to accelerated bone loss, which explains why osteoporosis, the world's most common bone disease, is rampant in postmenopausal women. Loss of bone mass accounts for the prevalence of hip and vertebral fractures as well as the hunched-over posture of many older women. All women should be particularly aware of the natural measures needed—and available—to prevent this crippling disease.

Clearly, estrogen is vital to the female body. When we produce too much or too little, symptoms occur. However, even though more than fifty symptoms have been attributed to the endocrine changes that occur during the climacteric—such as tiredness, nervousness, headaches, irritability, depression, insomnia, joint and muscle pains, dizziness, heart palpitation, breathlessness, and impatience—a direct cause-and-effect relationship for each one has not been clearly determined. Ovarian decline and diminished estrogen levels are hardly the only factors to consider when it comes to menopause. More important may be the overall health of the individual and her ability to adapt to all the various transitions taking place in her organ systems.

Physical Changes Following Menopause

* Some atrophying of vagina, cervix, uterus, and ovaries takes place.
* Vaginal wall shortens, thins out, and loses muscle tone.
* Labia majora become thinner, paler, less elastic.
* Supporting structures lose muscle tone (sphincter muscles, bladder, rectum).
* Secretion of cervical mucus is reduced.
* Breast size, firmness, and shape changes.
* Body hair gets thinner in most; in some, it increases.
* Wrinkling and loss of skin tone occur.
* Body fat is redistributed.
* Bone mass is lost.
* Metabolic rate becomes slower.

The following chapters discuss specific symptoms and problems associated with menopause in more detail. Remember that, for the most part, suffering through severe symptoms is neither normal nor necessary. In most cases, a commonsense approach to nutrition, regular exercise, and an otherwise healthy life-style are the only "medication" you need. It's all up to you.

Chapter 3

—— ❧ ——

Hot Flashes

A flush is anything but a flash.
—John W. Studd, MRCOG
King's College Hospital, London

The most characteristic complaint of menopause is the bothersome hot flash, more correctly called hot *flush*. Up to 80 percent of women suffer from them to some degree. Hot flashes may begin when periods are still regular or are just starting to fluctuate, and are often one of the first indications that menopause is approaching. Generally, hot flashes are most uncomfortable in the first and second years after menopause, gradually decreasing in frequency and intensity as the body adapts to the hormonal changes. Some women never have a hot flash, while others are inconvenienced for as long as five or even ten years.

Medical textbooks describe hot flashes as the result of *vasomotor instability*, a condition that affects the nerve centers and the flow of blood. The hormonal changes taking place in the menopausal body cause the blood vessels to dilate (enlarge) and constrict (narrow) irregularly and unpredictably. When they dilate, the blood flow to the skin, brain, and vital organs increases, and a sensation of heat covers the entire body. It usually starts in the face and neck and works down to the chest. The face may turn bright scarlet and the woman may perspire easily, or not at all. In some cases, chills will precede or follow a hot flash. Flashes differ in duration and frequency. Usually an episode lasts two to three minutes, but it can extend up to half an hour. Some women experience the sensation several times a day or night, others only once or twice a week.

The hot flash is harmless; nevertheless, as the body's temperature control system vacillates between overheating and recooling, a strain is put on other body systems as well. When flashes occur too often, they may be accompanied by side effects such as fatigue, weakness, dizziness, headaches, or loss of sleep. The lack of sleep may not appear serious at first, but over a period of time it can lead to depression, sexual problems, lethargy, and other psychological manifestations.

WHAT CAUSES HOT FLASHES?

The hot flash is still not fully understood; researchers have only recently determined that there are measurable hormonal changes during a hot flash. Earlier, flashes, like so many menopausal symptoms, were regarded as a figment of the female imagination—at least the medical community takes this phenomenon seriously now. The current consensus is that vasomotor instability is related to an increase in the levels of the two brain hormones, FSH and LH. These hormones directly affect the muscles that constrict and expand the blood vessels; thus, the higher the levels of FSH and LH, the more the vessels expand, carrying more blood and raising the temperature of the body.

The entire biochemical story is not quite this simple; however, nothing in the body ever is. The hyperactivity of ancillary glands involved in the endocrine upheaval may also contribute. Penny Budoff, M.D., believes that the release of other hormonelike chemicals called prostaglandins may affect the dilation of blood vessels, as well.(1) Clearly, more research is needed if we are to understand fully how a hot flash occurs as well as the method for treating it.

WOMEN MOST LIKELY TO HAVE HOT FLASHES

The fact that hot flashes are somehow related to changing estrogen levels is undisputed. An abrupt drop in estrogen tends to lead to more severe symptoms; a gradual decline causes fewer annoying flashes. Women with more body fat encounter fewer problems; small, thin women complain more frequently. Women who have had their ovaries surgically removed or have suffered damage to these organs also demonstrate greater susceptibility to hot flashes. And smokers can expect to suffer more than nonsmokers because smoking reduces hormone output and inhibits circulation.

You don't have to be menopausal to experience a hot flash. Waves of heat may hit anyone, at any age, caused by behavior that forces the heat-regulating system to step up its activity. Such behavior may include eating too fast, eating heavily spiced foods, exercising (especially if you are not in condition), rushing around, vigorous lovemaking.(2) In sensitive people, hot drinks, warm weather, too much caffeine or alcohol, marijuana, sugar, drugs, or stress may disturb the temperature-regulating mechanism in the brain, cause dilation of the blood vessels, and bring on hot flashes.

TREATING HOT FLASHES NATURALLY

Treatments that stabilize the autonomic nervous system (which controls our involuntary responses) may help bring hot flashes under control. Regular and moderate exercise, for instance, will decrease FSH and LH levels, reducing or even eliminating symptoms.(3) The hypothalamus, located in the brain, regulates the menstrual cycle, body temperature, and the autonomic nervous system. During menopause, when the hypothalamus becomes supersensitive to outside signals, exercise can stabilize it and help to restore more normal hormonal levels.

Exercise is considerably more effective, however, if it is begun well in advance of menopause. If your body is not conditioned, exercise may stimulate the very mechanism you are trying to suppress. Keeping the body in good working order also enables it to handle any discomfort with greater ease.

Proper nutrition can help in preventing and treating hot

flashes. Hormones are formed from the building blocks of food, and if even one nutritional element is missing, a hormonal deficiency or imbalance may result. Prevention of any physical ailment is always preferable to curing it; thus, nurturing the organs and glands throughout life with the right foods should be our primary goal.

"Accentuate the positive, eliminate the negative" is the basic formula for a healthy life—and it is crucial for the menopausal woman. For example, it is common knowledge that women share a health hazard—a penchant for sweets. Every school function, church social, and office meeting involves cream-laden pastries and coffee (double trouble). Too much sugar can be dangerous at any time; when hormones are erratic anyway, we must be exceptionally disciplined in this area. London University's Dr. John Yudkin, in his book *Sweet and Dangerous*, warns against the ill effects refined sugar can have on the hormones. A high-sugar diet, he reports, "can cause a striking increase in the level of adrenal cortical hormone . . . it can slow the rate of transport of hormonal chemical by as much as two-thirds even in one week."(4)

Blood-sugar imbalance, or hypoglycemia, is clearly a factor in women who experience hot flashes.(5) Hypoglycemia is now called idiopathic postprandial syndrome (IPS) by the medical community. If your first menopausal symptom is a hot flash, consider: How many of the known triggers of both hot flashes and hypoglycemia—caffeine, alcohol, heavily spiced foods, sugar, and so on—are a normal part of your diet? Write down what you eat for one week to find out. The cookies and doughnuts are obvious, but how much sugar do you put in your coffee? How many colas do you gulp down between meals? Are you drinking three glasses of wine at each meal and then ending with dessert? Do you overeat? Many sugar-filled items are easily overlooked, for example, many condiments that you normally add to your foods contain relatively large amounts of sugar (catsup, salad dressing, relish, tartar sauce). Cumulatively, they may be weakening your adrenal glands so that estrogen is not being converted efficiently. They also put stress on the pancreas, which results in fluctuating blood-sugar levels.

NUTRIENTS THAT SUPPRESS HOT FLASHES

Clinical studies have shown certain nutrients to be effective in treating hot flashes. The most widely researched is vitamin E. Tests indicate that when vitamin E is insufficient, the levels of hormones FSH and LH increase.(6) Since these hormones already tend to be overabundant in menopausal women, a shortage of vitamin E could exacerbate the situation. In women, vitamin E appears to have a stabilizing effect on estrogen levels, increasing the hormone output in women who are deficient and lowering it in those who are prone to excess. Adequate doses can buffer the hormonal ebbs and flows during the change, relieving associated symptoms. Other menopausal symptoms that are helped by supplemental vitamin E include nervousness, fatigue, insomnia, dizziness, heart palpitations, and shortness of breath.(7)

Many nutritionists agree that the increased prevalence of refined foods, coupled with the absence of whole grains, nuts, and seeds in the diet, has led to a dangerous decline in dietary vitamin E. To compound the problem, vitamin E is destroyed when exposed to the air, heated, frozen, or stored. While minor shortages rarely degenerate into a classic "deficiency disease," weakness on the deeper, cellular level makes us susceptible to a host of symptoms, some of which appear to be directly related to menopause.

For relief of hot flashes, Barbara and Gideon Seaman recommend starting with 100 IU of vitamin E, gradually increasing the dosage over a period of a few weeks to a few months until you experience results.(8)

Don't be shocked if it takes 1,200 IU before any real reduction in the frequency or intensity of the flashes is apparent. Vitamin E should be complemented with the mineral selenium. Studies show that the two operate synergistically: their combined effect is greater than the effect if each were taken separately.

As a fat-soluble nutrient, vitamin E is absorbed from the intestinal tract and only in the presence of fat. To ensure absorption, take vitamin E with a meal incorporating some fat—not, for example, with grapefruit and coffee. You can also aid its digestibility and utilization by taking it with lecithin, which is a fat that has been reported to reduce hot flashes effectively.

Note: If you have high blood pressure, diabetes, or a rheumatic heart condition, please do not take more than 30 IU of vitamin E without first checking with your physician.

Additional nutrients beneficial in minimizing hot flashes and stabilizing the endocrine hormones include vitamin C (combined with equal amounts of the bioflavenoids) and calcium.

In the mid-1800s, Lydia Pinkham concocted a vegetable compound to cure female maladies. For more than 100 years, her company continued to sell this natural remedy as an alternative to medical prescriptions. Since the days of Ms. Pinkham, women have passed down tried-and-true herbal remedies. Until recently, modern medicine held that these recipes merely provided a placebo effect for the hysterical woman captive to her hormonal fate, but no longer. Herbs that were at one time considered worthless are now being studied and tested for the treatment of every known ailment.

Not surprisingly, the herbs found most effective for menopausal complaints are quite similar to those contained in Lydia Pinkham's original formula. These herbs, known to be natural sources of estrogenic substances, act on pituitary and adrenal glands to stabilize the menstrual cycle. They include fenugreek, gotu kola, sarsaparilla, licorice root, and wild yam root. Nan Koehler, a botanist and herbalist, suggests making a tea with one of these herbs combined with another herb high in minerals, such as dandelion leaves, alfalfa, or borage.

Ginseng, a particularly potent herb, has been known and studied for 5,000 years. In several countries it is used to correct any type of temperature imbalance, such as chronic sweating, heat stress, or hot flashes. It, too, is said to exert a "normalizing" action on the pituitary gland, as well as help in rebuilding tissues, stimulating energy, regulating blood pressure, and generally rejuvenating the body, strengthening it against the debilitating effects of stress.

It is available in many different forms: instant teas, powders, capsules, and concentrates. Both Chinese and Korean ginseng are considered top quality. As a supplement, it is probably easiest to take in capsule form.

Correct ginseng dosage varies with body weight. If you weigh between 100 and 130 pounds, take 1,000 mg daily, half before breakfast and half in the middle of the day. If the capsule is measured in grains rather than milligrams, 8–10 grains converts to approximately 500 mg. Unlike most vitamins, ginseng is most effective when taken on an empty stomach, not with meals. It is best not to take it with vitamin C, since ascorbic acid tends to neutralize its value. So far, none of the tests to which modern scientists have subjected this ancient herb have shown it to have a single deleterious side effect.(9)

WHERE DO I START?

If you are bothered by incessant hot flashes, start by eliminating those foods that are obvious triggers. Check your diet to see if you are promoting blood-sugar imbalances. Fasting all day and overindulging at night can be just as devastating to the body as gulping down four cups of coffee and two chocolate-filled croissants. Check to see if your diet contains adequate amounts of the nutrients mentioned in Appendix C. If not, add more foods that incorporate these nutrients to your menus or supplement as indicated. It is better, when supplementing, to try one nutrient or herb at a time so as not to overwhelm the body. Also, that way, if you have any kind of allergic reaction, the source will be obvious.

Remember that your body is unique, and your program will be unique also. Just because vitamin E worked for your friend doesn't mean it will remedy your flashes. In his book, Dr. Atkins recounts the determined endeavors it took to find the right natural remedy for various patients. "While vitamin E in 800 IU worked for one woman, another tried vitamin E, diet, ginseng, dong quai and still didn't feel better until lecithin was added to her regimen."(10)

Natural Remedies for Hot Flashes

* Exercise moderately and regularly.
* Eliminate triggers: sugar, coffee, alcohol, spicy foods, hot drinks, warm clothes.

* Keep your blood-sugar level constant.
* Include of or more of the following to your diet:
    * vitamin E (800–1,200 IU, divided 1 to 3 times daily, mixed tocopherols preferred)
    * selenium (15–50 mg)
    * lecithin (6–12 capsules, divided 1 to 3 times daily)
    * vitamin C with bioflavenoids (1–3 gm spread throughout the day)
    * calcium (1 gm)
    * herbs: fenugreek, gotu kola, sarsaparilla, licorice root, wild yam root, dong quai
    * ginseng (1,000 mg, divided twice daily)

Chapter 4

———— ❧ ————

Insomnia

The best cure for insomnia is to get a lot of sleep.

—W. C. Fields

The inability to fall asleep and stay asleep is a major problem for many menopausal women. Nightly hot flashes, physical discomforts, changing life patterns, and emotional uncertainties all contribute to this condition.

The seriousness of insomnia is often minimized. We all know that in the short term it can leave one tired, emotionally drained, irritable, and anxious. Over a longer period, persistent sleeplessness can lead to far greater psychological problems: depression, disorientation, inability to function, even paranoia, uncontrollable rages, and hallucinations. The problem must be dealt with as soon as it is recognized.

While it is tempting to rely on sleeping pills, these are probably the worst choice in the long term. Sleep-inducing drugs change normal sleep patterns, and often exacerbate rather than cure the problem. And though they may provide relief initially, after a few short weeks, an increase in dosage is usually required—and we are all familiar today with the addictive nature and unhealthy side effects of these drugs. According to Quentin Regestein, M.D., writing in a highly respected medical journal, "Chronic use of sleeping pills does not get the patient to sleep any faster, but rather increases nightly awakening, abolishes deep sleep, and may continue to affect sleep patterns for five weeks after drug withdrawal. . . . the patient relying on hypnotics is often left with his original insomnia plus a drug problem."(1) Why take the risk when natural remedies have proven so effective?

NATURE'S REMEDIES

There are many natural, effective ways to promote sleep. The oldest is probably a glass of warm milk. With heat to quicken digestion and calcium to soothe the nerves, warm milk at bedtime should be enough to send most of us straight to dreamland.

Milk also contains a natural tranquilizer, tryptophan, in small amounts. This amino acid (one of the building blocks of protein), also found in turkey meat, is a precursor of serotonin, an important neurotransmitter associated with moderating pain, relieving depression, and regulating sleep. Administration of tryptophan at bedtime has been reported to improve the pattern of sleep in people who have insomnia. Research done by A. J. Cooper in 1979 concluded that this one amino acid significantly decreases the time necessary to fall asleep, increases the duration of sleep, and perhaps even improves the quality of sleep.(2) Extremely effective for most individuals, tryptophan is virtually without side effects, as it is rapidly metabolized by the body.

While it is best to derive nutrients from food sources whenever possible, to use tryptophan as a sleep aid may not be possible—one would have to consume an enormous amount of milk or more turkey than one's stomach could comfortably hold. In order for tryptophan to pass the "blood brain barrier" it must have no competitors, and milk or other protein-rich foods contain several other amino acids as well. Increased intake of this one amino acid is best accomplished by taking a supplement of L-tryptophan (1–3 gm) after a meal high in complex carbohydrates.(3)

Certain nutrients seem to work well when combined with L-tryptophan. Vitamin C, inositol, and vitamin B-6 promote sleep with or without the help of the amino acid. Inositol, sometimes found in lecithin, may also be taken separately in doses of 1–2 gm. Niacinamide likewise enhances the action of tryptophan. In some people, it has antianxiety activity of its own, and may help to reduce some of the nervousness that keeps many women awake.(4)

Magnesium relaxes the entire nervous system; thus, a woman who is extremely anxious, constantly agitated, and unable to relax or sleep may be getting a message from her body that she needs more magnesium. Researchers have discovered that a low level of magnesium is one of the unexpected consequences of rigid dieting. When women cut calories they tend to avoid high-mineral foods: whole-grain breads and cereals, beans, and nuts. However, taken in small portions, these nutrient-filled foods will not add fat to the body, and they may be helpful for relaxation and sleep.

Many teas have been promoted by different cultures for their hypnotic potential. These include hops, passion flower, catnip, basil violets (the leaves), lemon verbena, and the most popular, camomile. Lawrence Gould reports, "Ten out of twelve patients fall into a deep slumber shortly after drinking camomile tea."(5)

EXERCISE TO SLEEP

There is another treatment for insomnia—exercise. Vigorous physical activity reduces stress, relaxes muscles, and facilitates sleep. It also changes the quality of the sleep. The restorative, deep sleep that we all require can be increased by just 30 minutes of exercise three times a week.

Exercising for sleep works better if you are already physically fit. An Australian scientist reported in 1978 that when fit and unfit people exercised, the amount of slow-wave sleep (quality sleep) increased in the fit people but not in the others.(6) Even on days they did not exercise, the physically fit individuals had relatively more slow-wave sleep.

For exercise to be effective as an aid to sleep, it shouldn't come too close to bedtime. A morning aerobics class is more likely to produce refreshing sleep at night than a jog around the block late in the evening. Remember that exercise speeds up the metabolism, and it stays up for at least one hour.

HELPFUL HINTS

There are certain obvious techniques—tricks, if you will—that can be used in conjunction with natural remedies to help you relax and thus sleep better.

* Cut down on high-stress foods: french fries, colas, concentrated sugars. They elevate blood fat levels, blood pressure, and resting pulse rate, and they keep you hyped up.

* Do not eat a large meal less than four hours before bedtime. Digestion interferes with sleep.

* Try a long, tepid bath. Lock the door, take the phone off the hook, and if family is around, ask not to be disturbed. Breathe deeply while you are soaking. Concentrate only on inhaling and exhaling. This is a fantastic tension reliever.

* If you are upset, write it down or tell someone. Don't try to sleep with unexpressed anger.

* Sex to some women is a precursor of sleep, to others it is not. Know how it affects your body and tell your partner, so there are no hurt feelings.

* Start a regular exercise program today.

Natural Remedies for Insomnia

* L-tryptophan (1–3 gm if necessary)—best combined with a high-carbohydrate meal
* calcium (1–2 gm)
* magnesium (500 mg–1 gm)
* camomile tea

Chapter 5

―🐝―

Fatigue

Female fatigue is the most common "Silent
Disease" of women.
　　　　　—Elizabeth Weiss, *Female Fatigue*

How often do you say that you feel tired and listless, that you lack
vitality at the end of the day? Such complaints come not only from
menopausal women but from many women over 30. What is most
exasperating is that, in the majority of cases, doctors report no
physiological basis for these symptoms. Boredom, stress, depression, and psychosomatic tendencies are often suggested as explanations for fatigue. This may very well be true, but let's consider
some other, equally valid possibilities.

　　Energy levels depend on many factors, some psychological,
some physiological. Three culprits stand out among the physiological causes of chronic fatigue:　low blood sugar, anemia, and
underactive thyroid. Each condition can be the result of several
factors; the most likely but least considered are usually the nutritional ones. In other words, these conditions can be created and
treated by the foods we eat or don't eat.

　　Remember, as our organs age, they are no longer as resilient
as they were when we were 20. Many foods that we once devoured

with relish gradually become toxic to our bodies. Our glandular system needs to be treated with respect; our days of indulgence diminish with each passing birthday.

BLOOD-SUGAR IMBALANCE

Almost all of us experience either the late-morning or the mid-afternoon "droops" and regard it as a normal part of our daily routine. If we haven't eaten in several hours, it is not especially surprising that we feel tired and weak, have a headache, can't think clearly, lose our tempers, and crave sweets. We may be inclined to ignore these symptoms, but we should not. Our body is communicating something to us: we are being warned of a metabolic imbalance that, left unchecked, could lead to far greater problems.

The metabolic imbalance to which I refer is called hypoglycemia, or, more commonly, low blood sugar. Hypoglycemia results from an imbalance in the body's sugar-regulating mechanism that prevents the maintenance of a stable level of sugar in the blood. The body breaks down carbohydrates (starches and sugars) into glucose, the fuel on which we operate. If too much glucose is circulating in the body, the excess is taken out of the blood with the help of hormone insulin and is stored in the liver as glycogen. As the fuel is used up in daily activity, glycogen is gradually converted back into glucose, thus maintaining a stable blood sugar level.

When the system is flooded with sugar, this equilibrium is disrupted and the body goes into a tailspin. Nearly every organ and gland has to work overtime in a furious attempt to bring the blood back to normal. For a while we feel high, ready to take on the problems of the world, but the elation is short-lived. The pancreas, reacting to what it perceives as an emergency, pours extra quantities of insulin into the bloodstream, which withdraws the sugar from the blood and restores equilibrium. In its exuberance, the overcompensating pancreas usually withdraws too much sugar, causing the blood-sugar level to drop dangerously low. What we now experience is fatigue, weakness, shakiness, loss of coordination, headaches, hostility, and a craving for more sugar. To ease these unsettling feelings, to "calm our nerves," we usually grab a cookie, cola, cigarette, or cup of coffee. This may provide momentary relief, but the pancreas overreacts again, the cycle continues, up and down, day after day, year after year. Ultimately, the glands and the organs weaken.

Eating too much sugar is probably—no, definitely—the greatest offense we women perpetrate against our bodies. Whenever we're bored, anxious, happy, or depressed, we eat. Even those women who restrain their urges three weeks in the month may succumb two days before their periods and head straight for the nearest chocolate bar. It is not surprising that we suffer anxiety mixed with fatigue when we choose to subject our bodies to this roller-coaster existence.

There is a common expression male gynecologists use to describe the turbulent feelings supposedly experienced by women in connection with various life cycles and menstrual events: "raging hormones." This absurd expression has been used to explain and/or dismiss all female complaints. While our hormone levels do vary at different stages in our lives, whether or not they "rage" may relate to factors other than the female cycle. It is just as likely that a blood-sugar imbalance resulting from stress or improper diet could be causing hormone instability. If this is the case, then men, like women, can also suffer from uncontrollable "raging hormones"—or mood swings.

A woman may experience fatigue caused by a blood-sugar imbalance even if she is not a diagnosed hypoglycemic. Low blood sugar is relative; even if a person falls well within the normal range (60–120 mg) on a glucose tolerance test, she may experience symptoms. Barbara Edelstein, M.D., finds that when blood sugar drops suddenly, even though not to a critical level, some women get very anxious, some burst into tears, some feel shaky, and some become confused.(1)

Other conditions that can precipitate blood-sugar imbalances include severe and prolonged stress, pregnancy or lactation, cancer, tumors, chronic infection, and glandular malfunction. So be on the alert if any of these conditions describe you.

For the most part, hypoglycemia is self-induced. By persistently eating highly refined carbohydrates such as white sugar and white bread, drinking endless cups of coffee, and smoking cigarettes, we upset the blood-sugar mechanism, forcing it out of control. Years of abusive behavior render many of the endocrine glands ineffective. As a result, the adrenal glands, the pituitary, the pancreas, and the liver may all produce decreased amounts of hormones no matter how much they are stimulated. Eventually, even minor stresses (large helpings of cake or ice cream) turn into major events as the body, worn out from misuse, either refuses to respond or overreacts.

The human biochemical system is not adapted to handle concentrated sugar. Not only is refined sugar devoid of any nutritional value, it leaches the body's vitamin and mineral reserves in the effort to digest it. All carbohydrates require certain nutrients in order to be metabolized, the most important of which are the B-complex vitamins. Without adequate amounts of these vitamins, sugar ferments in the digestive tract, where it is later converted to acetic acid and alcohol. Thus, too much sugar coupled with too few B vitamins results in overacidity, gross nutritional imbalances, and low blood sugar.

This is not to say that I advocate a lifetime without chocolate cake. I am not suggesting complete self-denial. Such a program is extremely difficult to maintain in the long run, and unless you are very highly motivated or have a serious illness, chances are you will fail. Realistically, if you can get by without sugar for five days out of seven you are doing very well; six days out of seven is excellent. Remember, the older your body is, the less able it is to bounce back from dietary indiscretions. So, be good to yourself—decrease your intake of sugar and increase your ratio of good to not-so-good days.

One more tip about sugar. On the days when you cannot resist that special treat, supplement with a B-complex vitamin. It won't balance the scales completely, but the ill effects will be reduced and symptoms will be more moderate.

Many of us who were brought up on dessert after every meal have a hard time believing that sugar is all that harmful. The facts, unfortunately, are clear. Refined carbohydrates in general, and refined sugar in particular, have been implicated in a wide array of health problems, from obesity, diabetes, coronary thrombosis, and tooth decay to high blood pressure, menstrual cramps, premenstrual syndrome, cancer, and mental disturbances. In countries where people live primarily on whole foods, many of these problems are absent. When refined sugar and refined carbohydrates are introduced to these countries, however, the "diseases of civilization" emerge within ten years.

The constant need for sugar has been compared to addiction. William Dufty, a self-proclaimed former "sugar addict," writes in his book *Sugar Blues* that the only difference between a sugar habit and narcotic addiction is one of degree: "Sugar takes a little longer, from a matter of minutes in the case of a simple sugar like alcohol, to a matter of years in sugars of other kinds."(2) This may seem like a bit of an exaggeration, but try going two days without your nightly raid on the refrigerator or your afternoon pick-me-up, and then think about it.

If you have the symptoms listed below, you need to be particularly cautious about the amount of concentrated sugar you consume, and if you feel you can't possibly give up sugar, I urge you to read Bill Dufty's book. His personal story of how he kicked his "habit" is fascinating, and his practical instructions for change are most helpful.

Your body is always giving you signals, telling you when something is not working correctly. Fatigue is only *one* of the warnings of an erratic blood-sugar level. Some others are listed below.

Symptoms of Low Blood Sugar

* sudden feelings of nervousness, a sensation of "going crazy"
* periods of irritability for no reason
* spurts of energy after meals, followed by quick exhaustion
* sudden feelings of faintness or dizziness
* periodic bouts of depression
* sudden headaches
* temporary feelings of forgetfulness and confusion
* unprovoked anxiety and worry

* feelings of internal trembling
* heart palpitations
* rapid pulse without exercising
* abnormally antisocial feelings
* indecisiveness
* crying spells
* unexplained phobias
* frequent nightmares
* cravings for sweets
* indigestion, gas, colitis

Hypoglycemia is a disease with many causes, including a number of genetic, functional, or dietary imbalances. Because it is known to imitate other disease states, a comprehensive examination and a six-hour glucose tolerance test are essential for identifying severe problems. It is best to look for a nutrition-oriented physician or nutritionist because many orthodox physicians are not trained to recognize nutritional imbalances. Dr. Richard Brennan, founder of the International Academy of Preventive Medicine, claims that "despite hypoglycemia's seriousness, nine out of ten physicians who come in contact with the disease misdiagnose it."(3) Most physicians do not treat the problem, they treat individual symptoms. Often, and I think this is especially true in the case of women, they dismiss the patient as a hypochondriac.

Please don't misunderstand. I am not anti-medicine. Clearly, in order to have a disease diagnosed and treated, you must see a medical doctor. The point I am making is that most physicians are not trained to recognize and treat nutritional problems, and there *are* problems caused by bad nutrition. So, if your doctor is unable to find a functional disturbance and your symptoms persist, consider seeing a nutritionist.

Sugar is not the only factor to consider if your blood-sugar level is erratic. There are several other triggers of which you need to be aware. Coffee, chocolate, cola, and certain teas all contain caffeine, which plays havoc with the body's sugar mechanism. Caffeine stimulates the adrenal cortex to produce more adrenalin, which in turn induces the liver to break down glycogen into glucose. Many people are unaware that caffeine is hidden in many soft drinks and in common over-the-counter medications such as Anacin, Excedrin, Midol, and appetitie suppressants.

Alcohol, too, provides a temporary spurt of energy, quickly followed by a letdown. Physicians who have studied alcoholism believe that hypoglycemia may be a prime causative factor in this addiction as well.(4)

Cigarettes are now known to change the rate at which the body handles food. A clinical experiment found that women who smoke more than fifteen cigarettes a day are apt to be fatigued as a result of the amount of nicotine their bodies are required to metabolize. Although the harmful effects of smoking can be partly offset through nutrient supplements, it is far better to put an end to the habit. In preparation for quitting smoking, you can fortify your body by taking the following daily: a high-potency multiple vitamin and mineral tablet; : vitamin C, 1–3 gm; vitamin E, 400–1,000 IU (dry form); selenium, 50 mcg 1–3 times; and cysteine, 500–1,000 mg. In addition, take vitamin A, 10,000 IU, daily for five days, then stop for two.(5)

Stress in any form—physical, emotional, chemical, or nutritional—overworks the adrenal glands and can, therefore, bring about blood-sugar imbalances. Since we cannot avoid all emotional stressors, and most of us cannot escape environmental chemical stresses, we should learn to deal with those conditions over which we do have control—the physical and nutritional factors. We can physically strengthen our bodies through exercise and nourish them with food and supplements, tipping the balance in favor of regeneration rather than degeneration.

Blood-sugar imbalances can be controlled through a dietary program that reestablishes biochemical balance. Since many factors can raise or lower the blood-sugar level, it is important to treat the whole person. Each person's needs will be different; minor imbalances can be controlled by altering the diet, but in extreme situations, heavy nutrient supplements may be needed.

To reverse high blood-sugar levels and to relieve fatigue, your diet must be designed for a slow release of insulin from the pancreas. This, in turn, will ensure a steady release of glucose into the blood throughout the day. The foods to emphasize for such a program are protein (meat, fish, cheese, seeds, and nuts) and complex carbohydrates (vegetables, beans, whole grain breads and cereals, and some fruits, depending on the severity of the problem). Small, frequent meals are recommended, as well as the elimination of concentrated sugars (even fruit juice, for sensitive people), caffeine, cigarettes, marijuana, and certain medications. This diet, by the way, is recommended for everyone, not only for people with blood-sugar imbalances.

Eating properly may not be enough for a person with a more severe imbalance. Physicians who treat hypoglycemia find that between-meal nutrient supplements must be included. People whose diets have been deficient in vitamins and minerals, amino acids, and unsaturated fatty acids for years require greater than standard amounts of these nutrients in order to reverse the negative hypoglycemic cycle.(6)

The inability to handle stress and an uncontrollable desire for sugar are major factors in the development of hypoglycemia. Both conditions quickly burn B vitamins, leaving the person devoid of energy. A B-complex vitamin supplement can compensate for this deficiency. I recommend a formula that contains 10–20 mg each of vitamins B-1, B-2, B-3, B-6, and 100–250 mg of pantothenic acid. Additional sources rich in B vitamins include desiccated liver, wheat germ, and brewer's yeast.

A variety of nutrients participate both directly and indirectly in maintaining blood-sugar balance. Without the complete array of nutrients, glandular functions are diminished and hormonal output becomes erratic. For example, it is known that hormones from the adrenal cortex are very sensitive to a vitamin A deficiency. If adequate vitamin A is not available to the gland, then cortisone, the adrenal hormone that balances the effects of insulin, will not be synthesized.

You may be eating foods with vitamin A and still be deficient. While the vitamin does occur in large amounts in carrots, liver, sweet potatoes, and other green and yellow vegetables, many people have difficulty converting carotene (the form of vitamin A found in vegetables) into the usable nutrient. In that case, supplements may be indicated. An appropriate range for most adults is 5,000–20,000 IU.

Vitamin C is also important in the utilization of sugar. In 1977, Dr. Fred Dice of Stanford University reported that the dose of insulin required to control the sugar level in a diabetic who lacked the ability to produce the hormone was cut in half when the patient took high doses of vitamin C.(7)

The ability of Vitamin C to produce energy and reduce fatigue has been noted by many scientists. How it accomplishes this, however, is not really clear. It is thought that vitamin C cleanses the body of pollutants and blocks the formation of carcinogens found in foods and in the body. It also may prevent "tired blood" (blood that is low in oxygen, thereby slowing down its energy-producing functions) by increasing the production of leukocytes (white cells that fight infection) and hemoglobin (red blood cells that carry oxygen to all the cells). Without this important vitamin, energy-giving iron would be ineffective. Whatever the scientific reason, vitamin C works to conquer fatigue, as indicated in a study in which more than 400 people were interviewed. Those who took more than 400 mg of vitamin C per day clearly experienced less fatigue than did the people who were not supplementing.(8)

The minerals magnesium, potassium, and chromium are all involved in the metabolism of carbohydrates; thus, they affect energy levels. Magnesium sparks more chemical reactions in the body than any other mineral, and an undersupply of magnesium can cause fatigue, weakness, and irritability. Potassium deficiency is capable of causing symptoms similar to those of low blood sugar. This was brought to public attention when American astronauts made one of their first lunar flights. They suffered heartbeat irregularities because the synthetic orange juice they were given to drink lacked potassium. And finally, chromium, too, has been shown to be indispensable to the production of insulin and to the metabolization of glucose. Chromium is best taken in a brewer's yeast product that contains the chromium compound called glucose tolerance factor (GTF). This form of chromium is more easily absorbed and is better at stabilizing blood sugar than a standard chromium supplement.

Supplements That Aid in Balancing Blood Sugar Nutritionally

* multiple vitamin/mineral supplement
* B-complex vitamins (10–29 mg), 3 times daily for extreme cases
* pantothenic acid (100–250 mg)
* vitamin A (5,000–10,000 IU)
* vitamin C (50–500 mg)
* magnesium (500 mg)
* chromium (200 mcg)

ANEMIA

Amemia is a reduction of the amount of hemoglobin in the blood and/or a reduction in the number of red blood cells themselves. In either case, the reduced amount of oxygen available to the body cells causes decreased efficiency of body processes. The brain reacts to the lack of oxygen with headaches, dizziness, a feeling of faintness, loss of memory, nervousness, irritability, and drowsiness. Other danger signs are rapid heartbeat, numbness and tingling in the fingers and toes, ringing in the ears, black spots in front of the eyes, and a craving for ice, dirt, clay, or laundry starch.

Anemia is never a disease in itself, but is always caused by other factors. The change in red blood cells may be due to the use of certain drugs, exposure to certain insecticides, infection or disease, endocrine disturbances, or bone marrow atrophy. Usually, however, anemia results from either chronic blood loss or a lack of adequate nutrients, most notably iron.

Since more than half the body's iron is present in the red blood cells as a component of hemoglobin, any blood loss results in iron depletion. Hemoglobin, the protein that transports oxygen from the lungs to the tissues and cells, not only houses the iron, but depends on it for its production. Even something as innocuous as hemorrhoids or ulcers can cause enough blood loss to deplete iron stores. Anyone who continually loses blood obviously requires more iron.

During her childbearing years, a woman's requirement for iron is greater than a man's because she loses blood each month.

If she has profuse or prolonged periods, or if she is using an in-trauterine device (IUD), chances are she may be losing consid-erably more iron than is safe. For example, IUD users are apt to develop iron deficiency because they lose up to five times the amount of blood that other women do during menstruation.(9)

Inadequate iron in the blood is a very real problem in both young and middle-aged women. Many studies reveal that the vast majority of women take in only one-third to one-half their total daily requirement. The reasons for this are twofold: they are not consuming enough iron-rich foods, and the iron in the foods they are eating is not being utilized completely by the body.

It is difficult to eat adequate amounts of foods containing iron. Unless you love liver and can handle several cups of beans a day, you're not likely to make the 18 mg RDA (recommended daily allowance) through diet alone. To combine foods high in iron is possible; unfortunately, not only would it require time and careful planning, but the amount of food needed would exceed 3,000 calories daily. For many women, the time, bother, and possibility of weight gain are just not worth it.

Even if you did make the effort to eat the required amount of iron-rich foods each day, you would still have to take into account the fact that iron is poorly absorbed by the body. According to most textbooks, only 10 percent of the iron ingested is used by the body. For those who want to try to take care of their need for iron through their diet alone, I offer some advice. When it comes to ab-sorption, the very best source of iron is liver. The other sources (spinach, peanut butter, legumes, nuts, wheat germ, molasses, apricots, and raisins) need nutritional assistance to do the job. Dr. James Cook, director of hematology at the University of Kansas Medical Center, suggests that if you combine grains, vegetables, and dried fruits with vitamin C, you can increase iron utilization as much as fourfold.(10)

Certain chemicals found in foods diminish the absorption of iron. Tannic acid (found in many teas), phytic acids (an ingredient in grains and cereals), and phosphates (a preservative added to most packaged bakery products, ice cream, and soft drinks) great-ly decrease iron utilization.

Another problem relating to increased iron need is occurring since women are exercising more. Iron is lost in body excretions, such as sweat. Therefore, if you have frequent and strenuous workouts, you may lose significant amounts of sweat as well as significant amounts of iron. If you do exercise regularly, make sure your diet is generous in iron or take supplements.

Many women require iron supplements. There are a variety of sources to choose from, and it is hard to know which is best. All of the ferrous compounds are good (ferrous gluconate, ferrous fumerate, ferrous peptonate) except one, ferrous sulfate, which destroys vitamin E.

Vitamin C is helpful for the absorption of iron and certain other minerals (especially calcium, copper, cobalt, and manganese) should also be present for optimum effect. Usually, if you are eating a well-balanced diet or are taking a multiple vitamin/mineral tablet, these "micronutrients" are included.

Anemia and fatigue can be caused by a deficiency in nutrients other than iron. Lack of either folic acid or vitamin B-12 may produce fatigue, as well as symptoms such as apathy, withdrawal, and slowed mental ability. Like iron, folic acid is involved in creating normal red blood cells. A deficiency causes fewer cells to be produced, which means less hemoglobin and eventually less oxygen to all the cells. Folic acid deficiency is common in women, especially in women taking or making excess estrogen, pregnant women, alcoholics, and the elderly. Folic acid and vitamin B-12 interconnect biochemically, therefore they are best taken together.

Nutrients Beneficial for Treating Iron Deficiency Anemia
* vitamin B complex
    * vitamin B-1 (10–20 mg)
    * vitamin B-6 (10–20 mg)
    * vitamin B-12 (10–100 mg)
    * folic acid (0.4–20 mg)
    * PABA (up to 50 mg)
    * pantothenic acid (up to 100 mg)
* vitamin C (50–500 mg)

* vitamin E (25–500 IU)
* iron (18 mg)

HYPOTHYROIDISM

As your own medical Sherlock Holmes, consider one more condition that can cause chronic fatigue before, during, or after menopause. Hypothyroidism, or an underactive thyroid, means that the gland is producing smaller than normal amounts of thyroid hormone. This is another condition that may be quite widespread, yet frequently remains undetected. Yet there is no need to wait until symptoms reach dramatic, measurable proportions; early, subtle complaints may be clues enough. Fatigue is one of several indications of an underactive thyroid gland. Other symptoms include susceptibility to infection and disease, menstrual disorders, low body metabolism, unexplained weight gain, sensitivity to cold, constipation, loss of hair, dry skin, puffy eyes, and numb hands and feet. Obviously, these indications are general and could represent a number of problems. If you suspect they apply to you, however, follow up with self-help tests and, if indicated, check with your physician.

The symptoms of hypothyroidism are very similar to those of hypoglycemia. There is a logical explanation for this. According to Broda Barnes, M.D., a well-respected doctor who has published more than a hundred papers on the thyroid gland, there is a direct correlation between an underactive thyroid gland and blood-sugar imbalances; in fact, a drop in blood sugar is one of the symptoms of hypothyroidism.(11) As Dr. Barnes explains, when the thyroid is underactive, the liver is unable to release its stored glycogen and produce glucose, thereby causing a low blood-sugar condition. This theory has been tested in the laboratory. It has been noted that when the livers of laboratory animals are removed, blood sugar declines rapidly and death from hypoglycemia occurs unless glucose is injected intravenously.

Dr. Barnes suggests that both hypoglycemia and hypothyroidism can be diagnosed at home. In the case of hypoglycemia, simple observation of symptoms is sufficient. To detect an underactive thyroid, take your basal body temperature (the temperature of the body at rest) before arising in the morning. If it reads below 97.8 degrees, there is reason enough to suspect a thyroid deficiency. Repeat this for three or four days to be certain of your reading. (For accurate basal temperature measurement, before you go to sleep, place a thermometer by your bedside. As you are awakening, place the thermometer in your armpit and keep it secure there for ten minutes. Menstruating women note: It is best to take your temperature the week of your period, since temperature is more subject to fluctuation during the remainder of the month.)

Good nutrition contributes to the optimum functioning of all glands. For a healthy thyroid, however, the mineral iodine is at the top of the list. Deficiency of or an inability to metabolize iodine results in an enlargement of the gland, a condition known as goiter. Sometimes a sore neck will indicate a possible glandular dysfunction.

The most important dietary source of iodine is iodized salt. The concentration of iodine used in salt is one part sodium or potassium iodide per ten thousand parts of salt. If you buy iodized salt and use it in cooking or sprinkle it on your food, there is little chance that you need more. However, if your salt is not iodized or if you eat primarily cafeteria food or processed food, you run the risk of being iodine deficient.

Iodine cannot be presumed to be available in a "normal" diet. For example, while the daily requirement of 150 mg can be easily obtained by eating saltwater fish or seaweed, one would have to eat two pounds of eggs, six pounds of meat, eight pounds of cereal or nuts, or ten pounds of vegetables or fruit to reach this amount.(12) If you are not a fish lover, consider supplementing your diet with kelp tablets. One tablet four times a day will stimulate production of the thyroid hormone in most individuals. Remember that vitamin A and the mineral zinc must be present as well for iodine metabolization.

Lack of vitamin B-1 (thiamine) will eventually slow down thyroid function, and many of our everyday habits encourage this deficiency. Eating too much sugar is a primary reason for thiamine deficiency. The higher the sugar intake, the quicker and more intense the symptoms. Alcohol, coffee, and tobacco likewise eat up thiamine, creating what we commonly refer to as a "hangover," "coffee nerves," or a "nicotine fit." Everyday stress increases thiamine demand, and this includes the stress of exercise, so joggers, dancers, and aerobics freaks, beware.

When you are fatigued, the thought furthest from your mind is exercise, right? Right—and wrong. Try to overcome the urge to collapse; get out and do something. A brisk walk will stimulate your circulatory system and raise your metabolism. It might be a lack of physical activity that weakened your body's muscles and endocrine system in the first place. Oxygen is primary to every physical event in the body; a diminished supply results in a total degenerative effect. Exercise can specifically combat fatigue and increase your energy and endurance by forcing oxygen to your brain, heart, digestive system, and throughout your entire body.

One last comment concerning fatigue: Don't overlook the obvious. You may be overworked because you are trying to do too much, trying to be everything to everybody, and running yourself ragged. Think about it. Maybe your lack of energy is caused by to an impossible schedule. Examine your daily routine and responsibilities—you may need to look no further. A good source for more information about the so-called superwoman syndrome is Georgia Witkin-Lanoil's *The Female Stress Syndrome: How to Recognize and Live with It*.(13) Remember, workaholism is also an addiction—and a disease.

Nutrients Beneficial for Treating Hypothyroidism

* vitamin B complex (10–30 mg)
    * vitamin B-6 (10–30 mg)
    * choline (100–300 mg)
* vitamin C (50 mg–3 gm)
* vitamin E (25–300 IU)
* iodine (4 mg or 1 tsp kelp)
* vitamin A (5,000–20,000 IU) 5 times/wk
* zinc (15–30 mg)

Chapter 6

— ❧ —

Osteoporosis

What do menopausal white women, younger
women on contraceptive pills, diabetics, people on cortisone, smokers, the milk intolerant,
the aluminum factory worker, soda drinkers,
those who are sedentary, and those who prefer
steak-and-potato meals to eggplant casseroles
all have in common? Answer, a propensity to
osteoporosis.

—Betty Kamen and Si Kamen, *Osteoporosis*

THE SEVERITY OF THE PROBLEM

Osteoporosis literally means porous bones, or bones filled with tiny
holes. Clinically, it is not considered a disease per se, but rather the
progressive and severe loss of bone mass. Because of the loss in density, bones fracture more easily and heal more slowly as they
gradually waste away. To a limited degree, softening of the bones
is normal in both men and women of climacteric age; however,
weakness to the degree where you cannot function properly is not
normal, even though it occurs with frequency. For women, the loss
of bone begins sooner and proceeds six times more rapidly than it

does in men (primarily because women's bones are naturally smaller than men's bones).

Deterioration of bone density is the single most important health hazard for women past menopause—more common than heart disease, strokes, diabetes, rheumatism, arthritis, or breast cancer.(1) Half of all women between the ages of 45 and 75 show beginning signs of osteoporosis; one in three of these women have full-blown osteoporosis, and, by age 75, the number jumps to nine in ten for women with extreme bone deterioration.(2) Truly, this is a women's issue!

Osteoporosis is expensive. The average cost for two weeks of hospitalization after a hip fracture is roughly $10,000—and this doesn't include home care and rehabilitation expenses. In the United States alone, more than $1 billion is spent each year for the care and treatment of women with osteoporosis.(3) Similar costs prevail in the United Kingdom.

The severity of the problem cannot be overemphasized. Osteoporosis is painful and crippling. After menopause, a woman's the chances of fracturing a bone increase dramatically; even a minor fall or vigorous hug may precipitate a broken bone. Bone fractures characteristically result in immobilization, hospitalization, and dependence—taken to the extreme, even death. For example, hip fractures, one of the more severe consequences of weakened bones, are associated with long-term disability and an accelerated death rate. Between 15 percent and 20 percent of women die within three months of a serious fracture; about 30 percent die within six months either of the injury or of secondary complications, and those remaining are subject to recurring fractures or permanent disability.(4) The physical deformities caused by multiple fractures cannot be concealed: An older woman with advanced osteoporosis has lost height, is hunched over, has a protruding abdomen, and walks with a shuffling, unsteady gait. As the bones of the spine gradually lose density, the vertebrae collapse, forcing the rib cage to tilt downward toward the hip. A curvature in the upper spine (kyphosis) creates a second curve in the lower spinal column (lordosis), pushing the internal organs outward. The stomach protrudes so prominently that the woman may look as if she is in the sixth month of pregnancy. Because of the compressed spinal column, several inches in height can be lost (up to eight inches is possible) from the upper part of the body. The resulting "dowager's hump" is one of the classic stereotypes of aging—unfortunately it is not a myth (see Figure 5).

Internal functions are impaired as the compressed organs shift positions and obstruct other organs and systems. Constipation becomes a problem, and breathing may become labored. Aches and pains throughout the body, particularly in the lower back, may arise from pressure on the nerves emanating from the collapsed vertebrae. Life becomes a series of problems.

A woman's appearance and self-esteem may change drastically when osteoporosis reaches an advanced stage. Along with being uncomfortable and, to varying degrees, incapacitated, she tends to feel awkward, unattractive, and older than her peers. Her clothes don't fit properly anymore, and clothes shopping becomes

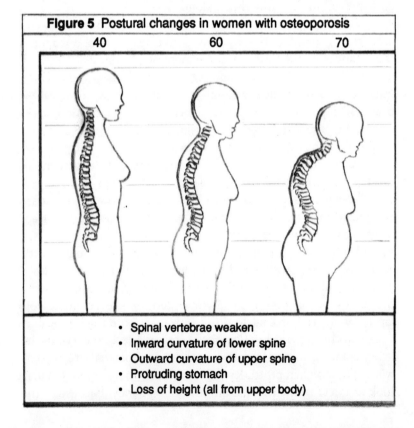

Figure 5 Postural changes in women with osteoporosis

40   60   70

- Spinal vertebrae weaken
- Inward curvature of lower spine
- Outward curvature of upper spine
- Protruding stomach
- Loss of height (all from upper body)

next to impossible as she tries to find garments that will mask her protruding stomach and slouching shoulders. Realizing that the body can never fully return to its premenopausal shape, many women with osteoporosis experience stress, anxiety, feelings of helplessness, and dread of the future. Psychologically, this loss of self-esteem and the emotional adjustments that must be made may be far greater problems than the physical inconveniences.

DIAGNOSING OSTEOPOROSIS

Diagnosing osteoporosis early is difficult because it produces no definitive symptoms until a fracture occurs. Usually, by the time bone loss is apparent through an X-ray, extensive and irreversible damage has already taken place. However, there are some early warning signs for which all women, especially menopausal women, should be alert: chronic low back pain, loss of height, nocturnal leg cramps, joint pain, transparent skin, rheumatoid arthritis, restless behavior (foot jiggling, hair twisting), insomnia, and periodontal (gum) disease.

A very controversial issue at this time is whether or not screening for osteoporosis is effective. Traditionally, one of the major problems in attempting to control bone loss has been the lack of sophisticated assessment tools for detecting early signs of bone demineralization. Whether or not the existing methods are useful for diagnosing the problem has yet to be determined. While opinions vary regarding the efficacy of osteoporosis screening measures as well as the best method of treatment, there is one point upon which most people agree, and that is the necessity of preventive measures.

CAUSE

Osteoporosis is a condition in which the reformation of bone has not kept pace with its breakdown or resorption. We usually visualize bone as a solid, rigid mass, but in fact it is an active, living tissue that, throughout life, is constantly being recycled. While the inner bone is breaking down, the outer surface is reforming. A delicate balance of the two processes is maintained constantly in response to the demands of the body. If the body needs calcium, bone is broken down; if it doesn't, bone is rebuilt.

When more calcium is withdrawn from the bones than is deposited, bones become soft and weak. Reversing this process is primary in preventing and treating osteoporosis. Confusion and conflict about specific recommendations arise because of the numerous factors that contribute to bone health; genetic predisposition, hormonal output, nutritional status, age, physical activity, and life-style habits. It is necessary to examine all the factors involved in this complicated problem.

WHO IS AT RISK?

One can never predict with complete certainty who will or will not develop osteoporosis, but there are enough clues so that probabilities can be drawn with a relative degree of accuracy. Let's start at the very beginning, with genetic inheritance. If a woman's mother, aunt, or sister incurred fractures because of weak bones, the probability that she may, too, is obviously great. I cannot agree, however, with those who believe that we have absolutely no control over inherited tendencies. Certainly, the weakness may exist; however, there is a host of information available to help compensate for genetics. That a woman's relatives had weak bones may indicate a family tendency toward osteoporosis, but it does not mean that she must suffer needless fractures. Her relatives may unknowingly have aggravated an already delicate condition. Were their diets poorly balanced? Did they suffer side effects from medication? Were they sedentary? Did they fail to exercise properly? As I will discuss in this chapter, nutrition and exercise are the keys to both preparing for and coping with osteoporosis.

Body size is a valuable clue to risk. Small-boned, thin women—women who wear petite sizes, or need to shop in junior departments—have a dramatically greater risk than larger women, simply because they have less bone to lose. Skeletal size, coupled with increased weight, helps explain why men and larger women are less susceptible to breakage. Bones respond to increased weight load by forming new bone tissue to meet the demand: the heavier you are, the greater the stress on your body and the more bone that is formed. According to researchers, the line of demarcation in terms of weight seems to be around 140 pounds; that is, those who weigh less than 140 have increased chances of developing osteoporosis. However, this should not be interpreted as an excuse for obesity, which carries with it far greater health risks than benefits. Exercise provides the same weight-bearing benefits as a larger body.

There are also racial differences in bone density and rate of bone loss. Black women appear to lose bone at a slower rate than Caucasian women. Weight is one factor, since black women at maturity generally have larger muscle and skeletal mass, but hormonal variations as well as skin pigmentation are also possibilities. It has been found that blacks have higher levels of calcitonin, a bone-protecting hormone, which enables their bones to utilize calcium more efficiently.

For some reason not clearly understood, the lighter the complexion, the greater the risk. This may explain the higher incidence of osteoporosis in Scandinavia and England than in China and South Africa. We should not, however, eliminate other possibilities, such as diet, physical activity, and hormonal differences among the races.

Women who undergo premature menopause (before age 45) have a more rapid decline in bone tissue than women who experience menopause naturally. The relationship between osteoporosis and estrogen became clearer during those years when hysterectomies routinely included removal of the ovaries. Surgeons now generally try to avoid removing the ovaries of premenopausal women to help prevent premature bone deterioration.

The building up and breaking down of bone is a complex process involving interactions of organs, hormones, and minerals. Any defect or disease that affects the nutrient transport system, endocrine, liver, or kidney functioning, or any illness that requires extended bed rest causes calcium loss and consequent bone loss. Anyone, of any age, who is restricted to bed rest for several weeks or more will lose calcium and bone at an accelerated rate.

Calcium metabolism is biochemically linked to carbohydrate metabolism. People who have diabetes or hypoglycemia are more likely to lose calcium from their bodies when their blood-sugar mechanisms are out of balance. Strict diet, nutritional supplements, and exercise are a must for these individuals.

Another major factor contributing to osteoporosis is a sluggish thyroid gland. Bone pain and spontaneous fractures can be manifestations of an underactive thyroid. Calcitonin, the hormone secreted by the thyroid gland, protects the bones from accelerated loss by enabling the calcium in the blood to be put back into the bones. A malfunctioning thyroid, unfortunately, will inhibit this building process.

Underactive thyroid function may be more widespread than was once believed. Dr. Howard M. Bezoza, an expert in the field of psychoneuroimmunology (which deals with the interaction of stress, hormones, biochemistry, and nutrition), analyzed his osteoporotic patients for thyroid function and found that more than 60 to 70 percent of the population over 50 is in need of thyroid stimulation.(5) Most likely, this problem develops slowly over time.

Are you at risk for osteoporosis? If you answer yes to two or more of the following questions, it is likely you are. The more risk factors that describe you, the more attention you should pay to preventive measures.

Are You at Risk?

* Has any member of your family had bone disease?
* Are you thin and small-boned?
* Are you fair-skinned?
* Were your ovaries removed before age 45?
* Are you childless?
* Have you been confined to bed for an extended time?
* Are you a diabetic or hypoglycemic?
* Are you lactose intolerant?
* Do you have an underactive thyroid gland?
* Do you have diabetes or kidney or liver disease?
* Are you sedentary?

* Do you avoid dairy products?
* Do you smoke cigarettes?
* Have you been involved in prolonged dieting or fasting?

THE ESTROGEN CONNECTION

Because of the correlation between estrogen decline and osteoporosis, estrogen replacement therapy (ERT) or the now more common hormone replacement therapy (HRT, which is usually therapy using a combination of estrogen and progesterone) is routinely prescribed at menopause in the hope of preventing further loss of bone. Does this mean that all women need to take estrogen before and during menopause to retain healthy bones? After 30 years of research, tests, and experiments, sharp disagreements still exist on this point among gynecologists, clinical orthopedists, and medical researchers.

There is no doubt that estrogen plays a primary protective role in preserving bone tissue. By allowing calcium to be absorbed more effectively and through other complicated hormonal processes, estrogen promotes strong bones. So what's the problem? What's the controversy? Those against ERT remind us of the possibility that, in susceptible women, estrogen replacement increases the risk of cancer of the uterus, hypertension, gall bladder disease, diabetes, and liver tumors. Whether or not it increases risk of breast cancer remains in question.

In a recent article in the highly respected *Journal of the American Medical Association*, a discussion of the pros and cons of ERT raised some cogent points: ERT does not result in replacement of lost bone tissue; when therapy is withdrawn, bone loss resumes.(6) The Boston Women's Health Book Collective adds to this, "sometimes at an even more rapid rate."(7) The implication is that once the estrogen treatment has begun, it must continue, not just through the menopausal changes, but throughout life.

Does this mean, then, that no woman should take estrogen even if she is a high-risk candidate for osteoporosis? No, it does not. When considering taking any medication, one must always weigh the risks versus the benefits. If your bone mass is low, as indicated by medical tests, or you have several of the risk factors listed above, the chance of bone loss may put you at far greater risk than would be posed for you by the use of therapeutic estrogen.

Estrogen replacement is *not* a desirable alternative for women with a history of uterine or breast cancer, high blood pressure, heart disease, blood clots in the veins or lungs, diabetes, stroke, liver disease, gallstones and gall bladder disease, migraine headaches, and large uterine fibroids. These women must seek other methods of treatment—and their numbers are large.

Current research suggests that when estrogen is taken in combination with its counterpart, progesterone, the risk of endometrial cancer is reduced; in fact, it is even lower than for women who take nothing.(8) During the menstrual cycle, progesterone is manufactured following ovulation; many of the risk factors for the development of endometrial cancer seem to be related to the long-term effects of estrogen unopposed by progesterone. Still, the effects of long-term use of progesterone are not known, and there are side effects of which women need to be aware. Progesterone can cause changes similar to those of diabetes, can alter blood fats unfavorably, and may stimulate the growth of breast cancer cells. If any kind of hormone therapy is used, very close follow-up is essential. Breast self-examination and sampling of the uterine lining must be done at regular intervals.

ERT and HRT are among the most controversial issues in female health care at this time. Those for and against these therapies offer sophisticated studies and logical arguments to support their opinions. The best a woman can do is stay informed, continue to question, and find out what best suits her needs. Whether or not hormones are indicated for you, diet and life-style are still important factors for preventing osteoporosis, and they have no negative side effects.

THE CALCIUM CONNECTION

The process that ends in osteoporosis begins 30 to 40 years before the first fracture. Bone deterioration can be controlled and somewhat reversed, but it takes time and patience. The longer you wait to take action, the smaller your chances of recovery. Prevention is the best—actually the only certain—course for maintaining bone health, and nutrition is the best alternative for retarding the demineralization of bone. And the story begins and ends with calcium.

The effects of calcium permeate the entire physical system. To say that calcium is important to the body is an understatement. Calcium is so vital to existence that a fluctuation of more than 3 percent in calcium level can result in severe debilitation and even death. Because calcium is instrumental in brain function, blood clotting, and muscle contraction, the body is equipped with an elaborate system of hormonal checks and balances to ensure that an adequate amount is circulating in the bloodstream at all times. When blood calcium levels fall, special hormones and glands respond immediately by withdrawing whatever is needed from the faithful storehouse, the bones.

An adequate amount of calcium in the blood is essential to maintain long-term bone health, so that continual withdrawal does not leave the body, decades later, with weakened bones. The latest recommended daily allowance of calcium for women prior to menopause is 1,000 mg; after menopause, 1,500 mg.

In preventing and treating osteoporosis, we need to consider three issues: (i) Are we getting enough calcium in our diets? (ii) If we are, what obstacles may be preventing us from utilizing the calcium for building bone strength? (iii) Is supplementation necessary?

Taking calcium into the body in the form of food should be a top priority, but there are factors that militate against it. Health professionals often fail to remember that many people either cannot tolerate dairy products or just don't choose to make them a part of their diets. For those who don't consume dairy products, alternatives include sardines (with the bones included), boiled turnip greens, and raw oysters. Now, be honest—how many times this week would you enjoy these foods? My favorite calcium foods are broccoli and almonds, but the amounts I would have to eat daily to reach the recommended requirements are totally out of sight. (For a quick check to see how much calcium you are getting on a day-to-day basis, consult Appendix C.)

And eating calcium-rich foods is only the beginning of the

story that takes calcium through the digestive system, into the blood, and finally to the bones. Numerous factors indicate that not all the calcium you take in is absorbed by the body; therefore, you may need even greater amounts of the mineral to compensate for the inefficiency. While absorption of any nutrient varies with the individual, at best, only 20 to 40 percent of the calcium you ingest is absorbed, and even that percentage decreases with age. Consider some of the complex aspects of calcium absorption:

* Your genetic makeup determines whether or not you are an efficient absorber.

* Disease or illness decreases the amount retained.

* Estrogen enhances calcium absorption, which helps explain the rapid loss of bone after menopause.

* Calcium absorption declines with increasing age in both men and women, but the decline comes earlier for women.

* Exercise increases absorption; inactivity decreases it.

* Medications, drugs, smoking, caffeine, and certain foods impede absorption, increase excretion of nutrients, and decrease utilization.

* Stress depletes your immediate supply as well as your storehouse of calcium if it becomes a chronic problem.

* Lack of other specific nutrients will deter absorption, especially vitamins D, C, K, and the minerals magnesium and phosphorous.

As you can see, drinking a glass of milk at night or popping your calcium supplement isn't enough to prevent or reverse the effects of bone loss. A total program is vital for those women heavily at risk.

Supplementation is a good starting point. There are many calcium sources on the market, and deciding which one to buy is the first step. Different tablets are derived from different sources, and some are combined with other nutrients for better absorption or because the nutrients work as a unit within the body. A calcium and magnesium combination is what I like best, because the two function together and are required by the body in a specific ratio. Of the calcium derivatives, calcium carbonate and calcium gluconate are among the more easily absorbed. While calcium carbonate is the most concentrated of the two, it can be constipating for some individuals; calcium gluconate is not. I do not recommend either dolomite or bonemeal; both were considered effective at one time, but new research indicates that dolomite contains the toxic metals lead and cadmium. Bonemeal is rich in the mineral phosphorus, which most of us need to minimize in our diets, not supplement. Phosphorus is part of the team necessary to calcium metabolism, but deficiency of the mineral is rarely a concern. Those who eat a typical modern-day diet including red meat, white bread, processed cheeses, soft drinks, and packaged pastries probably get too much phosphorus, because all these foods are loaded with phosphate food additives.

The proper ratio of calcium to phosphorus affects the amount of calcium absorbed by the bones. Ideally, the balance should be two to one in favor of calcium. With the abundance of phosphorus now found in foods, the balance has tipped in favor of phosphorus four to one. Not only is this change not conducive to calcium retention, it accelerates bone demineralization by stimulating the parathyroid glands, which secrete a bone-dissolving hormone called parathyroid hormone.

To reestablish the correct mineral ratio, reduce your intake of high-phosphorus foods drastically. Concentrate on eliminating processed foods that offer little nutrition anyway. These include almost all processed or canned meats (hot dogs, luncheon meats, bacon, ham, sausage), processed cheeses, instant soups, puddings, packaged pastries, soft drinks, breads, and cereals. Check the labels of packaged goods for ingredients such as sodium phosphate, potassium phosphate, phosphoric acid, pyrophosphate, or polyphosphate; if you find them, put the products back on the shelf.

Optimizing calcium retention requires adequate amounts of several other nutrients, including vitamins D and C and the mineral magnesium. A lack of vitamin D has been found in 30 percent of postmenopausal women with bone deterioration.(9)

Sunlight is the most effortless way to promote the manufacture of natural vitamin D in the body. Just 30 minutes a day of direct exposure is all that is necessary for the skin to produce the hormone. If this is not possible for you because of the climate where you live, or your life-style, you can get vitamin D from fatty fish (halibut, mackerel, salmon), fish liver, eggs, butter, and vitamin D-enriched milk.

The mineral magnesium is instrumental in converting vitamin D to its usable form and in keeping calcium soluble in the bloodstream. A magnesium deficiency disturbs the calcification of bone, impairs bone growth, and reduces calcium. Tests have shown that diets deficient in magnesium can lead to skeletal abnormalities, including osteoporosis.

Calcium, vitamin D, and phosphorus all increase magnesium requirements, thus emphasizing the importance of nutrient inter-relationships. Evidence suggests that the balance between calcium and magnesium is especially important. If the calcium level is raised, magnesium intake needs to be raised as well. The optimum calcium/magnesium ratio is two to one; thus, if you are taking 1,000 mg of calcium, you need 500 mg of magnesium.

Vitamin C is necessary for the manufacture of collagen, a fibrous protein that is found in connective tissue and cartilage, and is essential in proper bone formation. Since the need for collagen regeneration increases with age, vitamin C is also needed in greater amounts as one gets older. With age, the stomach tends to produce less acid. Vitamin C also facilitates the absorption of calcium by creating a weak acid medium necessary for proper digestion.

Nutrients Beneficial in the
Prevention and Treatment of Osteoporosis

* calcium (1,000 mg before menopause; 1,500–2,000 mg after)
* vitamin D (400–800 IU)
* magnesium (500 mg before menopause; 750–1,000 mg after)
* vitamin C (60–1,000 mg)

LIFE-STYLE FACTORS

The speed with which our bones break down depends on the way we treat our bodies: what we regularly put into them and how much we use them. Virtually everything we do can, in one way or another, be related to bone health.

A study of societies around the world has proven that specific diets show a direct correlation to advanced bone diseases. For instance, it has become apparent that a vegetarian diet helps prevent osteoporosis. Especially after the age of 50, heavy meat eaters lose almost twice as much of their calcium as do vegetarians. A number of medical investigators have found that consumption of high levels of protein, in excess of 120 grams per day, may stimulate bone resorption and encourage long-term bone loss.(10) One explanation is that meat is rich in phosphorus; the role of this mineral in causing calcium depletion has already been discussed. Another consequence of a high-protein diet is that it creates an acidity condition in the stomach that, over time, also results in bone resorption.

Protein, of course, is essential to health; but excess protein, especially in the form of fatty meats, leads to chemical imbalances and adverse symptoms. If you have been a heavy meat eater in the past, the risk factors for osteoporosis are stacked against you. I strongly urge you to deemphasize meat in your diet and to try eating more rice, bean, vegetable, and pasta dishes. Several Japanese and Mexican recipes, and vegetarian cuisine, offer a wide variety from which to choose.

Remember that both the amount and the *kind* of fat you consume affects calcium absorption. If fat consumption is too high or too low, calcium absorption is depressed. This has been a major criticism of reducing diets that call for nonfat milk and other fat-free products. Calcium requires the presence of some fat for its absorption, so for the sake of your bones you shouldn't eliminate all fat when you are dieting.

A certain amount of fat is needed every day for functions that cannot be performed by any other nutrient. Essential fatty acids (EFA) cannot be manufactured by our bodies and are necessary especially for the metabolism of calcium. The preferred forms of fat are those found in whole natural foods, such as whole milk, vegetable oils, and fish. Butterfat in fermented milk products such as yogurt and acidophilus are effective for encouraging calcium absorption. Even people who are sensitive to milk products usually can tolerate these because they are partially predigested. Include some in your diet daily.

The fats to avoid—those that alter digestibility and utilization of nutrients—are saturated fats (those that are solid at room temperature, like shortening) and certain vegetable oils, such as coconut or palm oil, found in processed foods.

Those of us with a penchant for sweets run a greater risk of developing osteoporosis. A high sugar intake encourages acidity, which causes calcium to be excreted from the bones. So, imagine the effects on your body of being both a voracious meat eater and a sweet-tooth fanatic!

There are a number of medications that interfere with calcium absorption. Some can easily be avoided; others cannot. If you must take any of the following drugs, consult your physician about the advisability of calcium supplementation:

* *Corticosteroids* (Cortisone, hydrocortisone, prednisone, and dexamethasone): Used extensively, these can cause severe bone porosity leading to ostporosis. They not only create a negative calcium imbalance, they also suppress the formation of new bone.

* *Anticonvulsants* (phenytoin, phenobarbitol, primidone, and phensuximide): These stimulate the production of enzymes that break down vitamin D, leading to deficiencies of both vitamin D and calcium, and, in turn, severe bone loss.

* *Antacids containing aluminum*: These cause an increase in calcium excretion. Aluminum-containing antacids do not cause osteoporosis per se, but they can be a contributor if taken on a regular basis. Check the label when buying antacids—or anything, for that matter. A few antacids that do not contain this element are Alka-seltzer, Bisodol, Eno, Titralac, and Tums.

* *Diuretics*: Many women take these to reduce blood
  pressure and body fluid. Some are thought to have an
  adverse affect on bone mass. During long-term usage,
  they may cause the blood calcium level to rise and
  excretion of calcium to fall. Morris Notelovitz, M.D.,
  director of the Center for Climacteric Studies in
  Gainsville, Florida, writes that Furosenide increases
  urinary calcium excretion, while Thiazide reduces
  the amount of calcium lost in urine, and thus is more
  appropriate for osteoporosis-prone women.(11)

Ask your doctor how your prescription drugs affect calcium balance.

To avoid the negative effects of diuretics, try reducing body
fluids by increasing foods that are high in water content: watermelon, parsley, celery, oranges, squash, and natural fruit and
vegetable juices.

Coffee, cigarettes, and alcohol also react negatively in the
body to produce bone porosity. It has been clearly established that
both heavy coffee drinkers and cigarette smokers lose more calcium from their bodies than nonusers. It is most likely that the acid
condition created by both is responsible for this. Decreased intestinal absorption of calcium is also related to alcohol consumption
and is much more pronounced in heavy drinkers. Frequent use of
antacids can further exacerbate this condition.

EXERCISE

Unlike ERT, or nutrient supplementation, there is no controversy
concerning the benefits of exercise in building and maintaining
strong bones. Like muscle, bone grows stronger with use. Bone
density depends directly on how much the bone is stressed. As
stress on the bone increases, the amount of calcium deposited in
the bones also increases. Bones of athletes and physically active
individuals are considerably heavier than the bones of those who
do not exercise.

No matter how old you are, exercise can strengthen your
bones. In a research project at Nassau County Medical Center in

New York, postmenopausal women who exercised for one hour three times a week not only stopped losing calcium but actually added some to their bones.(12)

It is never too late to improve the body. If you are not physically active at this time, start a program as soon as possible, if for no other reason than to protect your bones from deteriorating. The best exercises for bone strengthening are those that put a load of stress on your bones: jogging, aerobic dance, skipping rope, or brisk walking. To benefit fully, exercise for 20 to 30 minutes at a pace fast enough to accelerate your pulse rate moderately. For details on how to exercise properly, see Chapter 17. Any program of exercise or nutrition must be regular for optimum results, so working out four times a week is good; five times is better; six is excellent.

Frequently, women concentrate on aerobic exercises or exercises for the lower body and completely ignore the upper torso. This is why so many women have relatively weak arms and shoulders. For a thorough workout, put your bones and muscles through the full range of body movements. Walk or dance for the lower extremities, then add special arm and shoulder exercises, or work out with weights. Exercise physiologist Mary T. Lins explained to me that even a moderate weight-training program places repeated positive stress on the bones, thus increasing bone density.

To those of you who are conscientiously preparing for menopause by watching your food intake, supplementing appropriately, and exercising, a word of caution: resist going to extremes. We often mistakenly assume that if "X" is good for us, then "XX" is even better. Be moderate: exercise overdone can have a reverse effect on bone mass. Premenopausal women who exercise to the point of causing irregular periods or stopping them altogether begin to lose bone tissue. Why this happens is not clear, but researchers think that the loss of body fat experienced during long-term exercise programs alters hormone levels, preventing ovulation and the production of the hormones estrogen and progesterone. Also, because these women do not have much fat on their bodies, they are not producing the additional estrogen that is manufactured in the fat cells. The combined effect of the two processes is an abnormally low estrogen level, a factor known to accelerate the breakdown of bone tissue. If your periods are ir-regular or have stopped because of overexercising, you should reconsider your program. Your body is telling you something—listen to it.

Prevention is the best—and for some the *only*—way of avoiding the skeletal fractures, severe discomfort, and permanent disfiguration of osteoporosis. Once detected, osteoporosis can be controlled and reversed only to a limited extent, so the safest course is to begin now; exercise will add mass to your bones and years to your life.

Life-style Recommendations for Avoiding Osteoporosis

* Reduce red meat in your diet.
* Eat more cereals, grains, beans, pasta, vegetables, nuts, and seeds.
* Avoid foods containing processed fats.
* Minimize your intake of concentrated sugars.
* Reduce your intake of foods with phosphates.
* Stop smoking.
* Limit coffee, tea, and alcohol in your diet.
* Take drugs and medications only when directed and then only as long as needed.
* Take calcium supplements.
* Exercise, exercise, exercise.

PART II

Enjoying The Later Years

Chapter 7

❧

More than Skin Deep

I have some lines in my face from 50 years of
life. They tell me of years in the sun, of sor-
rows and joys. They tell me of time. They tell
me I have lived and that I am still alive. They
can't be erased. They can be softened. . . . Do
I long to be the smooth-skinned, freckle-faced
kid I once was? No. I long for the same thing
today that I longed for then: to be the best I
am able to be.

　　　　　—Kaylan Pickford, *Always a Woman*

How many of us are willing to admit that we don't always share
these lovely sentiments? As mature adults we would like to, but
looking into the mirror each morning to find pillow creases etched
on our cheeks, we wonder how long it will be until they last all day.
What cream can we purchase to smooth out the newly formed
lines? What miracle cure will erase these indelible markings?

　　The first visible signs of aging appear in the largest and most
public organ we have—our skin. A woman may feel young, think
young, and act young, but if her face is lined, society will remind
her that she has "crossed over" into middle age. And while men

seem to profit by their character lines and graying temples, signs of aging are not admired in women.

In the last several years, however, this attitude has started to change. More women are approaching the prime of life less panicked by a few emerging furrows. The time is coming when we will not only accept this change but consciously express the real beauty of the mature look.

So you should not be dismayed by aging skin—nor should you neglect it. No doubt, you want to look and feel as good as you can for as long as you can—and that is a function of nutrition and skin care. Knowing how our bodies change, and how those changes affect the skin, enables us to take necessary precautions to prevent premature wrinkling and maintain healthy skin tone. In this chapter I will provide long-range guidelines and specific remedies for healthier, younger-looking skin.

The way the skin changes depends partly on heredity and partly on a person's daily activities. All that we do to and for our bodies is eventually reflected in the skin, which is a mirror of our internal condition. If we choose to live in the fast lane, burning the candle at both ends—smoking, drinking to excess, eating junk foods, or worshipping the sun—we will definitely accelerate cellular destruction. On the other hand, if we avoid these excesses, or at least take necessary precautions against their effects, and concentrate on nourishing and rebuilding healthy cells, we can greatly extend our youthful appearance.

SKIN ANATOMY

The skin contains one-fourth of the body's blood supply, two million or so sweat glands, and even more nerve endings, hair follicles, and sebaceous glands. It performs many necessary functions: helping the body regulate temperature, eliminating waste products and toxins, and protecting the entire body from invading germs and harmful environmental conditions. It is an organ we must care for both inside and out.

Before we discuss skin-care techniques, however, we need to understand the life cycle of the skin. From the moment we are born, the skin is continually renewing itself. At any given time, approximately one-fourth of the cells are developing, one-half are mature, and one-fourth are in the process of degenerating. It is said that the human body gets a new outer skin every 27 days from birth to death. That means that what you are doing to or for your body today will show up in your skin next month.

There are three basic layers and several sublayers of skin, and it is deep within the body that a healthy skin is conceived. The underskin, filled with blood vessels, nerve endings, fat cells, hair follicles, and connective tissue, is the life-support system that transports nutrients to the visible external layer. Yet our outermost wrapping, or epidermis, the one we see each day, is often the only part of the skin to which we pay attention.

As we approach menopause, and even sooner for some women, several changes occur in the skin: the fat layer diminishes; collagen, the skin's structural support system, is produced in smaller amounts; and sweat glands function less vigorously. If precautions are not taken both internally and externally, a dry, sagging skin is likely to result.

Somewhere around age 35 external evidence of aging appears. Because skin cells are regenerating at a slower rate, as are all body cells, it takes more time for a fresh supply of cells to reach the surface. The dead outer covering that remains is now exposed to the elements for a longer period of time, resulting in a dehydrated texture. A general loss of oil and moisture make the skin thinner and less flexible. Dryness develops; fine lines and wrinkles emerge.

Men do not experience these aging conditions quite so early in life because normally their skin, is thicker. People with dark, thick, oily skin show fewer wrinkles than people with fair skin because the heavily pigmented outer layer protects the interior cells from the harmful effects of the sun. It also helps to remove the dead outer cells—as some men do by shaving. The practice of removing dead skin using a pumice stone or loofah, is helpful in creating a soft, smooth texture.

SKIN CARE IS MORE THAN SKIN DEEP

The condition of your skin is a fairly accurate gauge for determining how well you are treating your body. If you have been neglecting your health or have been under greater-than-normal pressure and tension, your skin will probably let you know. Fortunately, the skin will respond to any positive change in life-style more quickly than any other organ in the body. Learn how to deal with your stress; refrain from eating highly processed foods; stop smoking, drinking too much alcohol, and basking in the sun; feed your body with good, healthy food, and drink plenty of water, and see how your skin reacts.

All vitamins, minerals, and amino acids guard in one way or another against cellular destruction, premature aging, and, therefore, dry and wrinkled skin. The following list discusses these nutrients and their special roles.

Nutrients and Skin Health

* _vitamin A:_ keeps all tissues soft and healthy; guards against scaling and drying; acts as an antioxidant
* _B-complex vitamins:_ assist in tissue repair; prevent skin eruptions and hair loss; promote a healthy nervous system; improve circulation; regulate body secretions
* _vitamin B-6:_ aids in the utilization of DNA and RNA (basic to the process of cell reproduction)
* _niacin:_ improves circulation and reduces cholesterol; keeps skin, gums, and digestive tissues healthy
* _PABA:_ stimulates intestinal bacteria (used primarily as a sunscreen)
* _vitamin C:_ antioxidant; essential for healing and the formation of collagen; prevents capillary breakage
* _vitamin E:_ antioxidant; maintains healthy cellular respiration within the muscles
* _vitamin F (EFA):_ lubricates skin and hair; prevents dandruff, hair loss, and dry skin
* _iodine:_ essential for normal thyroid activity; necessary for skin, hair, and nails
* _zinc:_ forms collagen for binding cells together as tissues

* *iron:* vital for blood formation; a deficiency can cause dry skin

A healthy life-style is basic to healthy skin. Not getting a balance of nutrients or not getting enough nutrients can surface on the skin. Chronic dieters who are not eating adequate fat or protein often set themselves up for dry skin and dull hair.

Women who are eating adequately and still notice these conditions need to consider various possibilities. They may have a genetic susceptibility to skin and hair problems. They may have some other medical condition, such as an allergy, that could cause an outward reaction. They may be taking medication that produces changes in the skin or hair as a side effect. Or they may not be absorbing the nutrients their bodies need for a healthy appearance. For example, alcohol hinders the body's ability to absorb several of the B vitamins, and also disrupts levels of magnesium, potassium, and zinc. Foods high in saturated fats and concentrated sugars also demand greater nutrient requirements for absorption. When the diet consists primarily of these types of foods, there is a chance of undernutrition, which can show up on the skin.

METHODS OF SKIN CARE

Most vitamins and minerals need to be taken internally; some, however, can be applied externally. The B vitamin PABA (para-aminobenzoic acid) is considered the best protection against one of the greatest sources of damage to the skin, the sun. It is found in many popular sunscreens and should be used whenever the skin is exposed to the elements for any length of time. Since ultraviolet rays penetrate haze, fog, and clouds, PABA should be used even on overcast days or days when you cannot feel the heat. The amount of protection your skin requires depends on the type and color of your complexion. A fair, thin-skinned woman needs a high sun protective factor (SPF) of ten to fifteen. Darker, thicker skins can tolerate more exposure, and need an SPF of eight to ten.

Certain other nutrients can be used externally for various skin conditions. Vitamins A and D and zinc ointment are frequently used for dry skin and acne-related problems. These products can be bought over the counter in pharmacies and health food stores.

Many women ask if estrogen salve or cream will restore their youthful skin. It will, to some extent, but only temporarily. Initially, the hormone forces the skin to puff up with water and fat, but over an extended period of time it actually accelerates the breakdown of collagen fibers and blood vessels, thus hastening the loss of skin elasticity. Women using estrogen creams often complain of the same side effects as women who are taking birth control pills: skin discoloration, rashes, loss of hair, and oily skin. There are far safer methods to bring moisture to your drying cells.

ADDITIONAL FACTORS INVOLVED IN SKIN CARE

Any element that draws moisture out of the skin either internally or externally will result in drying and wrinkling. Be aware of aspects of your environment—air conditioning, steam-heating, and the sun, for example—that affect your skin, and take steps to minimize their dehydrating effects. Refrain from using harsh soaps and applying heavy makeup to the skin, since these, too, reduce natural moisture.

There are many ways to add moisture to your home environment. For instance, you can keep your bathtub filled with water when you are at home; the evaporation of water molecules moistens the air and hydrates the skin. Purchase a large aquarium, or fill your home with large plants and bouquets of flowers in oversized vases. In these ways you can enhance the loveliness of your surroundings while moisturizing your skin.

Adding moisturizer to your skin and protecting the innermost layers becomes more vital with each passing year. There are several safe products on the market that can plump up the tissue under the surface of the skin, smooth out already formed lines and wrinkles, and nourish beneath the external layers as well. Which moisturizers will work best for you? It depends on the ingredients and how sensitive your skin is. Don't assume that your moisturizer must be expensive. *Consumer Reports* tested 48 moisturizers and found that the most effective creams and lotions were the least expensive. Just look for the one with the fewest ingredients. The more ingredients in a moisturizer—perfumes, colors, thickeners, emulsifiers—the greater the chance of an allergic reaction.

At one time it was thought that skin creams did not penetrate the epidermis; however, now we know this is not true. Therefore, if you put anything on your face, check the ingredients to make sure there is nothing harmful in the product, such as alcohol, preservatives, fragrances, coloring, mineral oil, lanolin, and petroleum.

Skin-care product labels are often confusing; manufacturers are not required to list all ingredients or to indicate whether their sources are natural or synthetic. The use of synthetic ingredients, some of which are proven or suspected carcinogens (quaternium-15, formaldehyde, methyl- or propylparaben, hexachloraphene, NDELA [nitrosodiethanolamine], TEA [triethanolamine]), is especially problematic in lotions or creams that are designed to stay on the body for long periods of time (twelve hours). Immediate allergic reactions and irritations are obvious dangers, but what about the effects of continuous absorption of a potentially harmful chemicals over the course of several years?

Certain natural-product manufacturers have recently taken the initiative in developing safe skin-care products. A major improvement is the substitution of natural vegetable oils for mineral oil as the base of mass-market creams. Mineral oil, a petroleum derivative, is difficult to remove from the skin and can actually clog pores and cause blemishes. As it inhibits the ability of the skin to produce its own oils, it can worsen an already dry skin condition. Typical vegetable oils used are olive, wheat germ, safflower, sesame, almond, apricot kernel, and avocado, which are closer in composition to the natural secretions of the skin. Most of these oils are also rich in linoleic acid, an essential fatty acid that aids in skin cell renewal.

It also helps if synthetic coloring and scents are replaced with herbal extracts and powdered flowers. Some commonly used fragrances in natural creams include rose, iris, orange blossom, lavender, and camomile. Look for these ingredients on the label when shopping for face and body lotions.

Exercise is vital to vibrant skin and a healthy body. A strenuous workout will increase your circulation, enhance the absorption of nutrients, and stimulate the increase in collagen production. According to exercise guru Jane Fonda, "If your budget is limited, you'd do better to invest your money in a regular, sweaty, speed-up-your-heartbeat exercise program than in a lot of expensive hormonal creams, masks, facials, and the like, whose effect will be at best temporary and superficial."(1)

Many of the facial cracks and creases we develop are due less to aging than to habitual facial expressions and unconscious grimaces. Constant squinting, scowling, smiling, or frowning in time will leave permanent imprints on the face. To avoid this, some women have even learned to control their smiles. In a television interview, actress Morgan Fairchild demonstrated how she had taught herself to "laugh down" so that crows' feet and other laugh lines would not form on her face. I tried her exercise in front of a mirror and it wasn't easy, but if it is something you would like to explore, you can read about it in her book, _Super-looks_. On a practical level, I suggest you might try to avoid un-necessary squinting (especially when outside or reading), and to stop frowning. The furrowed brows and tight lips characteristic of scowlers are the most unpleasant of all permanent expressions.

CARING FOR THE REST OF YOUR BODY

So far, we have focused on facial skin, but we should not neglect the rest of the body. When it comes to total body relaxation, there is nothing that compares to a long, hot soak in the tub. Some experts claim, however, that baths are too drying for the skin, but I don't believe they need to be, as long as you moisturize afterward. Baths can be relaxing and invigorating for the body and the mind as well.

To make your bath special, add natural ingredients to the water for various effects. Cleopatra used milk in her bath; you might want to try adding a quart of milk to your bath water. For very dry skin, add one-half cup of sesame oil as well.

Some women like the fragrance and feeling that freshly brewed herbs offer. Brew your favorite combination (try rosemary, thyme, and lavender flowers) in a bowl, steep for about twenty minutes, strain and add the liquid to your bath.

If you are in the mood for an invigorating bath, if your muscles are aching from aerobics, or if you are tired or have a sunburn, try one cup of natural apple cider vinegar in your water. To really energize your body as well as your spirits, shower after soaking, alternating hot and cold sprays.

After soaking, use a loofah sponge to remove the dry, dead cells from the outer layer of skin. It, too, will invigorate you as it increases blood circulation and tones the skin.

HAIR

Hair is an extension of the skin, and it responds to changing hormones and normal aging in characteristic ways. Like the skin, hair reflects your state of health. Philip Kingsley, a British specialist in scalp and hair science, writes, "If you're not eating properly, or exercising regularly, or if you've been under a great deal of stress, the effects are bound to show up on your hair."(2)

Hair follicles are nourished deep beneath the surface of the skin, so if you have problems with dull, dry, or mousy hair, check your diet and daily habits before spending your entire paycheck on external conditioners and treatments. (External treatments need not always be expensive. They may enhance the hair's manageability and work with the nutritional treatments recommended here. For natural hair-care recipes, see Appendix D.)

Hormonal Changes and Hair Growth

At menopause, many women lose hair from all over their bodies. Some women, however, experience the reverse, and find hair appearing in places where they had never seen it before.

While facial hair may be unsightly or embarrassing, it is *not* a sign of emerging masculine tendencies. All it indicates is a reverse in the ratio of female to male hormones, both of which we all (men and women) share. Since estrogen is not dominant following menopause, the hair follicles tend to follow a male growth distribution pattern. Unfortunately, nothing has been found to reverse this hormonal process, and women plagued with unwanted facial hair have only cosmetic solutions. One alternative is bleaching the hair if it's dark; removal of the hair through waxing, depilatories, or electrolysis is another approach.

Nutritional Possibilities for Problem Hair

Sudden hair loss, or hair that is dry, greasy, or lusterless, may not always be hormonally related; it may be nutritionally induced. Healthy hair depends on a delicate balance of protein within the hair shaft and oil outside the hair shaft. If the follicles are inadequately nourished, any number of symptoms might emerge. For example, if your hair feels unusually greasy, it may indicate a diet too rich in animal fat. Eliminating red meat, butter, fried foods, and pastries from your diet may be all that is necessary to reestablish chemical equilibrium. Dry hair frequently responds to foods rich in B vitamins, vitamin E, vitamin A, and a daily dose (2 tsp.) of vegetable oil. Loss of hair may be checked by adding high-quality protein to and eliminating junk foods from your diet, and supplementing with iron and zinc.

Fasting and fad dieting over the years often lead to hair thinning and loss. Past years of depletion can intensify a woman's present needs for nutrients, so that she will need greater amounts of all vitamins and minerals than if she had been adequately nourished all along.

It is also quite easy to overlook certain nutrients in your diet. For example, a subtle complication of the vegetarian diet, especially one that does not include egg and milk products, is the lack of one amino acid, methionine.(3) Even a slight deficiency in this nutrient over a period of time may result in loss of hair.

Certain drugs, most notably birth control pills, have been implicated in hair loss. If you are taking hormonal drugs of this kind, it would be wise to increase your intake of foods containing sulfur, the B-complex vitamins, and zinc (see Chapter 16 for the pill users' supplemental program).

Stress endured over a long period of time or a sudden traumatic experience may cause sudden hair loss or scalp disorders. However, usually the hair will return to normal when the situation has subsided. You can aid the process by making your diet rich in B-complex vitamins, vitamins E and C, and folic acid.

The Bottom Line for Healthy Skin and Hair

* Avoid environmental pollutants (smog, sun) if you can.
* Don't smoke.
* Minimize chemical drinks (coffee, tea, cola, diet drinks, and alcohol).
* Drink plenty of water.
* Don't lose weight too rapidly (two pounds a week at the most).
* Eat high-quality protein and complex carbohydrates.
* Minimize your intake of excess oil, saturated fats, and hydrogenated spreads.
* Reduce sugar and refined and enriched flours and grains in your diet.
* Keep the air in your home moist (especially if you live in a dry climate, work in an air-conditioned building, or fly often).
* Supplement your diet, emphasizing antioxidants (Vitamins A, C, and E).
* Exercise regularly.

INTERVIEW: VERA BROWN

To learn about the natural approach to treating the external skin, I interviewed Vera Brown, noted beauty and skin-care expert, owner of Vera's Natural Beauty Retreat, and author of *Vera Brown's Natural Beauty Book*. At her retreat in Tarzana, California, we discussed the fundamentals that all women need to know to keep their skin young and healthy, as well as to meet the special problems that arise at menopause. Vera not only answered my prepared questions, she also offered her personal insights into the deeper concerns of menopausal women.

Linda: I know you work with many women over 50. When they come to you for skin-care advice, what is the most important information you give them?

Vera: I feel that self-esteem is one of the most important things for women to have going through menopause. Even if they don't look any different and are not gaining weight, they *feel* as if they are. They may be retaining water and having temporary discomfort, so they feel different. They may hate their bodies, hate what their bodies are doing to them, and hate the way they look or think they look. It is so important for women to do whatever they can to change this.

So many women I have met who are going through menopause are very unhappy with themselves. You can take a woman who has had a wonderful outlook on life and suddenly she becomes depressed. She feels she's getting older. She feels less feminine. She feels her skin doesn't look good, her body doesn't look good. When women think of menopause—and this applies even to the young women who begin menopause early—the word brands you, so to speak. You are now older; you are no longer young. Of course this is not true, but many think it is.

I believe when a woman starts the menopause, that's the time she should really start to give herself some strokes. The way you give yourself strokes is to be nice to yourself. Instead of looking in the mirror in the morning and being unhappy with what you see, change your outlook. Look at yourself and think how lucky you are to be alive. How wonderful it is that now we have information that tells you how to feel better and look better. Look at the people years and years ago who didn't know about nutrition and didn't have the vitamin therapy and all the advantages that we have now to help us look better. I tell women, instead of waking up with a negative feeling, count your blessings, count all the wonderful things that have been discovered that help us go through this change.

Now, that is not to say that skin care is not important—it is vitally important. When you are going through menopause, many changes take place in the skin. For instance, it has a tendency to become dehydrated. So a simple skin-care routine is also mandatory.

Linda: What is the most common mistake you find older women make when it comes to their appearance?

Vera: I see women going one of two ways. Some women change their hair color, put on way too much makeup. They're trying to cover up their age. The others go to the opposite extreme and don't do a darn thing. They are depressed, so why even bother? The hot flashes are making them crazy, they can't sleep, so forget it. I hear this all the time. Well, I don't like that attitude one bit. When I get women in my office like that, I take them by the hand and put them in front of the mirror and tell them to say some nice things to that lady.

One of the things I teach is that skin care isn't just applying one cream after another. It's closing the door in the morning and evening in your bathroom or bedroom or wherever you have some privacy to let that time be just for you. That is the time when you are going to do something only for yourself. Think about what happens to you during the day: You get up in the morning, get dressed, wash your face, eat breakfast, talk on the phone, make appointments, see people, and all your energy is going out, out, out. How many times a day do you sit down, take a deep breath, wash your hands, rub them together, bring the energy back into the face and do a simple skin-care routine? It may just be washing your face, but do it with love. Use loving strokes, bring circulation back into your skin. You will feel better and you will look better. It's the same principle as exercising. If you do even a small amount every day, you will benefit not only physically but emotionally as well. You are doing something for yourself.

I had a wonderful discussion in Hawaii with a Japanese man, and he told me that when you say, "Take care of yourself" in Japanese, it literally means, "Put your hands on your face." In other words, the hands bring energy back. That is why skin care is so important. That's why I suggest people have facials. You're completely putting yourself in someone else's hands. It's another person giving you energy.

Linda: If we don't like what we see in the mirror, where do we begin to make the changes? What's the first step?

Vera: Try to make changes inside yourself first. Perhaps it's your self-image, your thoughts, or your diet that need changing. You know, your thoughts are far more important to your looks than *any* amount of money you may spend. When you feel you want to improve your looks, don't begin by globbing on all kinds of makeup to make your outside look different. It won't change you on the inside. Be nice to yourself. Keep yourself clean inside and out.

Linda: Can we treat the skin externally to prevent wrinkles and lines?

Vera: There is really only one way the skin cells can be nourished and that is the same way all other cells in the body are fed; from the blood. However, recent research finds that there are specific ingredients normally found in the skin that can be absorbed from the outside, such as collagen, amino acids, and elastin. These substances, which can be manufactured in laboratories, do help to replace some of the natural elements that have been lost because of poor health or environmental irritants. They can also help speed up the production of new skin cells, thus making the skin appear more supple, softer, and healthier looking.

Linda: Isn't the outside skin basically dead skin?

Vera: Yes, that's true. And it is very important to slough off the top layer so that the new healthy skin can surface. We can help this process by using facial scrubs, masks, or, in more extreme situations, peels [a substance that peels off the top layer of skin].

Linda: We know that wrinkles are caused by loss of moisture in the skin. What is the most effective way of retaining moisture?

Vera: A combination of cream over mineral water is the most effective treatment for the fine lines. Mineral water first reintroduces moisture into the skin, then the cream seeps underneath the skin's surface and pushes out the indentations caused by dehydration. The cream also acts as a seal to keep in the moisture. Now, deep wrinkles you're probably going to have to live with, unless, of course, you have a face lift. Even then, the surgery is not permanent. After about five years you will need another.

Linda: I'm an advocate of the preventive approach in every area of life. How can we best prevent wrinkling?

Vera: Foremost is to stay out of the sun. The more sun you get, the greater the elastin breakdown, the component that keeps the skin flexible. It's important to remember that sun damage is cumulative and you can't repair damage to your skin already caused by the sun. If you are an outdoor person, take practical precautions, wear a visor or hat, cover up with a sunscreen, and minimize your direct exposure, especially between 11:00 a.m. and 3:00 p.m.

Linda: How much sun can we outdoor people safely take and still maintain healthy skin?

Vera: That depends on how fast you burn. But no one should be in the sun for any length of time. It has been proven that the sun rays are very harmful to the skin and body. There has been such a tremendous increase in skin cancer and melanomas. Next year, it is predicted that 500,000 people will contract skin cancer. So, when people ask me how long can they stay out in the sun, I tell them it depends on their sensitivity—some people should never go out in the direct sun. There are also many things you should not do in the sun: use perfume, drink alcohol, or take medications like diuretics, antibiotics, or hormones of any kind. Tetracycline and sulfa cause rashes if you are in the sun; cortisone can cause inflammation around the hair follicles; birth control pills and hormones can cause discoloration of the skin; and Valium can cause measlelike eruptions if the skin is overexposed. Many drugs and chemicals are photosensitive to the sun and will cause scales, pimples, or rashes on the skin.

Linda: Do you believe in exercising the facial muscles in any particular manner to prevent wrinkles?

Vera: I really don't believe in facial exercises. I have seen too many people who have overexercised a muscle or gotten poor results. Unless facial exercises are done under professional supervision, I don't recommend them. I do use massage and face acupressure (the application of pressure at specific body points) to increase circulation. [These procedures are illustrated in *Vera Brown's Beauty Book*—see the "Resources" section at the back of this book.]

Linda: Are there any other factors we can control that will prevent unnecessary skin aging?

Vera: Sure, I just mentioned that if you make the same face over and over again, you will develop permanent creases; well, this is certainly true of cigarette smokers. Over a period of years, lines form around the lips because every puff on a cigarette causes the muscles around the mouth to contract. More important, smoking reduces your oxygen level, which affects circulation—the primary source of nutrition for all cells. The smoke, too, dries the skin and deposits a film of tar and oil on top. So, stop smoking, if you can, and you will prevent a lot of unnecessary wrinkles.

As we all know, alcohol in excess impairs the functioning of the liver, which, in turn, affects every other organ in the body. It can contribute to broken or enlarged capillaries near the surface of the skin. You can determine if you are drinking too much if, when you look in the mirror, you see redness or blotchiness, particularly on the cheeks and nose; dullness or poor texture; and excessive wrinkles from the drying effect.

There are many other factors that we can sometimes control in our lives that cause the skin to lose moisture: chlorine in swimming pools (wash your face with water to dilute the chlorine as soon as you get out of the pool); smog, pollution, and wind (the best protection is to minimize exposure and use a good moisturizer, sunscreen, and mineral water); and air conditioning/heating (a light spray of water several times a day is great).

Linda: Are there any other situations of which we should be aware that can result in unhealthy skin?

Vera: There are so many. Stress obviously is a big problem but unfortunately no skin treatment—aside from massage—will alleviate it. It must be taken care of mentally, emotionally, and internally. Lack of sleep and overwork can cause poor color and texture and dark circles under the eyes. Poor skin color is the direct result of poor circulation. When the body isn't receiving its nutrients for whatever reason, the skin will mirror the problem. That is why it is also important to maintain your gastrointestinal system as well, if you want good skin.

Linda: What is a basic skin-care routine?

Vera: A basic skin-care program starts with a cleanser void of lanolin or mineral oil. You want to use a cleanser that penetrates the skin because the most important thing about skin care is to keep it clean. There is nothing more important. So many women who wear makeup just use soap and water to remove it, and they are not getting a deep enough cleansing. You need a cleanser that actually penetrates the pores. Scap does not. After cleansing, use a freshener, void of alcohol, to remove any residue left on the skin. Next, I suggest using some kind of a facial mist to return moisture to the skin. I have one that is made up of minerals and rose water, but mineral water will do as well. This step is especially important for dry skin. While the skin is still damp, you put on either your moisture cream (a.m.) or night cream (p.m.) and put it on sparingly, just a very little. You should not use a lot of cream, especially at night. So many women going through menopause have these extreme sweats; they put lots of cream on at night and all this does is treat their pillowcases. You want your pores to be clean. Let them breath. You know, you are constantly getting new cells. You slough off the old cells and make new cells. It's a cycle. But as one gets older, the whole cycle slows down. If your cells are clogged, it slows down even more. This is vitally important, when going through menopause, use less cream at night so your pores will stay open. Never go to bed feeling cream on your face. The steps, then, are: cleanse, freshen, mist, and moisturize.

Linda: What about makeup? Do we require more or less as we get older?

Vera: As you know, I'm not a makeup lady. I don't wear any myself. I feel the less you use the better. I have lines in my face; I should, I'm 65. Now if I put a foundation on, it will accentuate the lines. So, I suggest, as you get older use less makeup and, if you can, use none at all. I am a firm believer in makeup for the eyes and lips but not the face.

Linda: Doesn't makeup give you some protection from the sun and other environmental elements?

Vera: No. If you have your face cleansed thoroughly and use a good moisturizer, you will get all the protection you need. If you go in the sun you must add to that a sun protector. As far as I'm concerned, makeup gives you no added protection. I know a lot of people feel that if they are in the sun all day they need the foundation, but I'll tell you what happens. When they sweat under a half inch of foundation, their pores get large because the makeup seeps into them.

Linda: I know you are a strong believer in facials. I've been under the impression that they are merely a luxury for the well-to-do. Are they all that important?

Vera: Yes. For most women, facials are the only truly certain way of achieving that deep cleansing that I mentioned. They also increase circulation and condition the skin. With commercial products, however, you may have to do some shopping around to find the right kind.

Linda: What if you can't afford a professional facial?

Vera: Then you should make an investment in products for the home. Maintaining a regular program on a daily basis will still give excellent results.

Linda: What are the basic products that a woman needs to promote and maintain her healthy skin?

Vera: Cleanser: purchase a cleanser with no mineral oil or lanolin, which clog the pores and are difficult to remove. If you use soap, it should be glycerin and without lye.

Freshener (also called toner or astringent): select one without alcohol or perfume. The acidity of the freshener will return your skin to its proper pH balance.

Moisturizer: again, read your labels and find a product devoid of mineral oil and lanolin. Best applied sparingly and followed by a spray of noncarbonated mineral water.

Masks: you can buy or make several kinds of masks. [see Appendix E for some natural recipes]. Before you do, though, determine what you want. Do you need deep cleansing, moisturizing, or peeling?

Scrubs: these are excellent for fighting blackheads, surface blemishes, and removing the ever-shedding top layer of skin. Some women use these once a week, others need it twice a week.

Linda: Is skin care any different for black skin?

Vera: For daily skin care, I treat black skin the same as white; the basic skin structure is the same.

Linda: Is there one last word you would like to give to women about to experience menopause?

Vera: Yes: Pay more attention to your appearance than you ever have before. You deserve all the loving strokes and tender loving care you can get. But you know what? You have to give them to yourself. This is a time when you should become very active. It's a time in life when the luncheons and shopping don't really fill the needs that you have. Go out and do things for other people. Get involved in a charity or anything. When depression sets in, the best thing you can do is to do something for somebody else. It works. You have to get up in the morning and have a purpose, especially at midlife.

You know the people that I've found who are hit the worst by this depression are extremely wealthy people. They've had no responsibilities. I tell them to get involved. When you get up in the morning have a purpose. Make each day count because every day is so beautiful. With all the heartache, sickness, and strife in the world, I feel that every day is a gift and we should cherish it.

Chapter 8

Sexual Changes

> With all the complexity, with all the difficulties, most midlife women will say; "Sex? It's gotten better and better."
>
> —Lillian B. Rubin, *Women of a Certain Age*

Menopause does not mean the end of sex. Quite the contrary; for many women, the midlife years are especially sexually satisfying and creative. Think about it: After nearly 40 years, you are free from the fear of pregnancy and the bother of birth control devices, tampons, and maxipads. What a relief! Better yet, opportunities that were few and far between when the kids were running in and out of the house are now available. An entire Saturday afternoon can be spent in a leisurely romantic interlude. You don't have to worry or hurry. Look forward to these days—they should be days of celebration.

Some of the hormonal alterations women go through at menopause actually heighten their sexual responses; some middle-aged women find sex more satisfying when they reach 50 than they did when they were 20. Those who imagine that women automatically turn into asexual beings at menopause should consider these revealing statements taken from *The Hite Report*.(1)

* "I believe sexual desire increases with age. Enjoyment certainly increases—I can vouch for that."
* "I didn't know getting older would make sex better! I'm 51 now and just getting started."
* "I thought that menopause was the leading factor in my dry and irritable vaginal tract. My doctors thought that it was lack of hormones . . . but with my new lover, I am reborn. Plenty of lubrication, no irritation."

Why do we expect the sexual charge to go out of our lives once we reach a certain age? I believe we are conditioned to expect this. All through life we are subtly—and not so subtly—indoctrinated by the media to believe that sex and beauty go with youth. The ads in any popular magazine show how true this is. So it is not surprising that many older women, when they spot a few lines on their faces and a few extra pounds on their figures, feel less desirable.

The emotional impact of these changes can be devastating for some women. Kaylan Pickford, a very successful New York fashion model who happens to be over 50 years old, observes that if a woman accepts the idea that only in youth is there beauty, sexuality, and therefore love, she falls into the trap of making unrealistic comparisons and becomes insecure. Pickford says that youth, middle age, and old age should never be compared. They are all as unique and beautiful as the changing seasons—each offers a fresh perspective, a different experience. To compare the first spring flowers with a summer sunset is ridiculous.

SEX: IS IT ALL IN YOUR HEAD?

"A woman's sex life after menopause is determined more by her psychological outlook than her physical changes (providing a dry vagina doesn't interfere with her sexual pleasure)," says Dr. John Moran, gynecologist and director of the Well Woman Centre in London. The fate of the libido seems to depend on a number of factors, such as individual genetic makeup, early childhood upbringing, and life experiences, all of which come into play long before menopause. Psychiatrists agree that the sex drive is predominantly psychological in origin, though controlled to a degree by the amount of steroids circulating in the blood. It is possible that women who complain that they do not "feel sexy" after the change did not feel that way before menopause. The very extensive Kinsey study found that some women use menopause as an excuse to curtail sexual relationships they were unenthusiastic about anyway.

To a large extent, however, how a woman responds sexually depends on the interest and response of her partner. Your husband, lover, or significant other may be going through his or her own midlife crisis. While middle-aged men do not experience the range of hormonal changes that women do, they do undergo anatomical changes that can reduce their sexual responsiveness. Like the woman's ovaries, the man's testicles decrease in size. The *vas deferens*, the narrow tube that transports sperm, becomes narrower, and the sperm become thinner and less plentiful. In terms of sexual response, it generally takes longer for them to reach arousal and orgasm. If the man is not aware that this is normal, he may become overanxious, and he may transfer his own insecurity to his partner. Researchers note that some women's psychological problems with sex during this time may be caused by men who, bewildered by their own changes in sexual performance, shift the blame to their partners.(2)

Around the half-century mark, men as well as women confront new problems and adjustments. They sometimes switch jobs, realizing that if they intend to make a career change it had better be soon. Children entering college may become a financial burden. Illness may enter people's lives, resulting in physical adjustments, economic insecurity, and emotional stress. The uncertainty arising from all these changes may be more responsible for sexual and marital problems than either hormonal or physiological changes.

It is said that the most difficult aspect of aging sexually is accepting it. Both men and women need to realize that all physical responses inevitably slow down. This has nothing to do with one's femininity or masculinity—it is normal. Allowing more time for sexual expression is important. The term *communication* often seems overused, but maybe that is because talking honestly about your troubles is good, commonsense advice. Share what is happening in your body with your partner, so that together you can creatively pursue ways of finding mutual satisfaction.

Myths and misconceptions have for too long defined sexual roles. For modern adult women, it is time to differentiate between the facts and the fiction. What do you know, or think you know, about aging, menopause, and sexual satisfaction that is real—and what is hearsay? Correct information is the best ally we have in preparing for the change—or any change, for that matter.

Physical Changes

The woman going through menopause experiences definite physiological changes in her female organs and hormonal secretions, some of which may result in a temporary decline in her sexual responsiveness. As Dr. Moran explained to me, "The dramatic change in hormone levels during the menopause accounts for a variety of unpleasant symptoms; chiefly, tiredness, lack of energy, low self-esteem, and poor memory. If the common vasomotor symptoms—hot flashes, headaches, and night sweats—are present, these can also lead to a feeling of being unwell. With all these symptoms, it is not surprising that sexual pleasure is diminished."

Losing sleep and finding oneself overtired is reason enough for anyone, at any age, to lose interest in sex. In time, many change-of-life symptoms do subside without outside intervention. The cessation of menstrual periods and declining levels of female hormones do not of themselves affect sexual desire. What few women understand is that the hormone most responsible for sexual arousal is the male hormone testosterone. Although testosterone is present in the female system prior to menopause, its effect is tempered by the larger proportions of estrogen and progesterone. As these female hormones decrease at menopause, the proportion of testosterone becomes greater. Indeed, there is increasing evidence that women's sexual interest and enjoyment do not fall at midlife, but rise because of the change in ratio of male to female hormones.

Declining hormone levels may not directly affect sexual response, but they do subtly alter the reproductive tissues, often leading to uncomfortable and even painful intercourse. The changes are usually gradual, different in each woman, and can be minimized and controlled by proper diet, regular exercise, and a healthy life-style.

The changes are most evident in the vagina, which becomes smaller, shorter, thinner, smoother, dryer, and less elastic. Because of the lack of vaginal mucus, a woman generally is slower to lubricate in response to sexual arousal. It usually takes a little longer for a woman to achieve orgasm, although, according to Dr. Niels Lauersen, gynecologist and professor of obstetrics at Mt. Sinai Hospital in New York City, the difference is not great—between seconds and minutes.(3) In any case, women need not feel insecure if they take longer to lubricate; remember that it also takes longer for the mature man to achieve erection. Actually, this is probably the first time in the sexual relationship where the time of arousal is close to equal—for men and women close in age, that is.

Other parts of the female anatomy also undergo minor changes. Like the vagina, the cervix, ovaries, and uterus diminish in size; the *labia majora* (outer lips of the vagina) become thinner, paler, and smaller; the breasts lose some of their fat, firmness, and shape, and may even become slightly less sensitive; clitoral stimulation may become irritating and annoying due to lack of lubrication. All of these changes are normal; some of them may be unnoticeable, others may be annoying, but they are easily treatable.

NATURAL REMEDIES

In a few women, decreased elasticity of the vagina along with the reduced ability to lubricate may cause vaginal dryness so severe that intercourse becomes uncomfortable or painful. In severe cases, it may even cause bleeding. The usual medical treatment is the female hormone estrogen. However, if estrogen is contraindicated for you or you would rather not take hormones, other, external, lubricants are available.

Aside from the old standby, K-Y Jelly, vegetable oil is also very effective. Do not use any kind of oil that contains alcohol, because it might irritate the genital mucus membrane. And do not use petroleum jelly (e.g., Vaseline)—it is not water soluble, and may get into the vagina or urethra, leading to irritation and, possibly, infection.

After menopause, the internal environment of the vagina changes from slightly acidic to alkaline. If you are taking estrogen or antibiotics, or overindulging in sugar and processed foods, this change may be even more pronounced. Coupled with the fact that the outer vaginal lips are now smaller and provide less protection for the vagina, urethra, and bladder, infections occur easily and spread quickly.

There are several natural solutions to maintaining and restoring vaginal Ph balance. Douching with a plain lactobacillus acidophilus yogurt is quite successful. Add a few tablespoons of yogurt to warm douche water, or, if you prefer, insert several teaspoons of yogurt into the vagina with a tampon and then lie down for five to ten minutes to allow time for it to work. (While you are relaxing, why not go ahead and eat the remaining yogurt? It functions even more effectively internally, to create a beneficial flora in the intestine.)

A woman's urethra is considerably shorter than a man's, and she is more likely to be bothered by bacterial infections. To prevent urinary infections, drink lots of water to flush bacteria out of the urinary tract. Plenty of cranberry juice also helps to restore the acid balance and retard further bacterial growth. Always empty the bladder immediately after sexual contact to keep unfriendly microbes from entering the urethra. And don't wear jeans, underwear, or pantyhose that fit tightly in the crotch. Buy cotton-crotch underwear so that the vaginal area is kept as dry as possible; bacteria multiply in a warm, moist environment. Finally, cut down on sugar and refined carbohydrates that drain your body of its disease-fighting nutrients, and make certain your foods are rich in vitamins A, B, C, and the mineral zinc.

Exercising the vaginal, stomach, and back muscles will greatly extend your years of sexual pleasure. Keeping all the muscles surrounding the internal organs toned and tight will prevent many common complaints, such as backache, fallen organs, involuntary urination, and excessive dryness. The most commonly recommended exercises are the Kegel exercises. Developed more than 40 years ago, they strengthen the pubococcygeus (PC) muscle, the band of tissue that extends from the pubic bone in front to the coccyx bone in back. Since the PC muscle supports the vaginal tissues as well as all of the internal pelvic organs, it requires continual strengthening.

Kegel exercises can be started when a woman is in her teens, although the better-late-than-never adage always applies. These exercises can improve sexual satisfaction and make childbirth easier. They are also useful for women of any age who suffer from poor bladder control and leaking urine.

If you are not sure where the PC muscles are, the next time you go to the bathroom, start and stop the flow of urine. The contraction you feel comes from these muscles. Try it without urinating. You will be able to exert even more pressure. You don't have to strain to gain benefit, so take it easy and be sure to continue breathing during the exercise. The Kegel exercises can be done anytime, anywhere, whatever best fits your schedule. And there are variations if you tend to get bored doing only one kind of exercise.

Kegel Exercises

1. Contract the PC muscle tightly and hold for 3 seconds, relax for 3 seconds, and repeat. Gradually build to 10 seconds.

2. Contract and release as rapidly as you can, starting with 30 and working up to 200.

3. A lying-down position works both the PC muscle and the internal organs. Lie down on your back, knees bent, with your feet on the floor. Raise the pelvis until you feel the pull and then begin squeezing.

Kegels are certainly the most popular exercises for strengthening and toning the vaginal muscles. We should not forget, however, other muscles in and around the reproductive organs that also require strengthening and toning. All of the muscles in front of, behind, and surrounding the female organs work best at protecting the lower body if they are tight and firm.

As with any other muscle, disuse of the vaginal muscle results in diminished tone and decreased flexibility, and eventually it atrophies. Many sex therapists recommend regular and frequent intercourse to ensure adequate lubrication, muscle tone, and continued sexual health. Ralph W. Gause, M.D. and sex therapist, observes that the decrease in estrogen and the lack of sexual activity work together. "The estrogen level may fall but if the vagina is sexually active, it remains fully functional."(4)

The enjoyment of sex has more to do with attitude and continued sexual practice than with all of the age-related changes mentioned. If you have had a rewarding love life before menopause, there is no reason to think that it will not continue. Should temporary symptoms arise, they can, for the most part, be treated with natural methods. A combination of a sound knowledge of the aging process, acceptance of yourself, and understanding toward your partner, will enable you to learn new, creative ways of finding sexual pleasure. If you honestly and openly try, the quality of your sexual experience will always improve with age.

HOW'S YOUR DIET?

A satisfying sex life depends on a healthy body. Both sexual function and desire are closely linked to hormone production and the condition of the endocrine glands. In order to function optimally, all the hormone-producing glands—including the thyroid, pituitary, adrenals, and sex glands—require nutritional support. Frequently, in cases of diminished sexual pleasure or arousal, the basic materials described below can reestablish sexual vigor.

Zinc, which is found in high concentration in the pituitary gland, is associated closely with blood histamine levels. Studies have shown that women with low histamine levels are unable to reach orgasm, whereas women with high blood histamine levels achieve orgasm easily. In men it is well established that the higher the histamine level, the quicker the ejaculation, and the lower the count, the slower the response. Men and women who take antihistamines regularly need to be aware of the possibility of decreased sexual desire, delayed orgasm, and ejaculation difficulties. Zinc deficiency is common in women because they lose significant amounts during menstruation. Diet often reinforces this loss. Refining grains and cereals removes 80 percent of the zinc in them, rendering these foods useless as sources of zinc. Foods from the sea, particularly clams, oysters, herring, and sardines, offer plentiful supplies of zinc, as do seeds and nuts, wheat germ, and wheat bran. If none of these is a regular part of your diet, I recommend that you take 15–30 mg a day of chelated zinc as a supplement.

Niacin, a B vitamin, is another nutrient that may be associated with histamine production. Life-extension researchers Durk Pearson and Sandy Shaw find that niacin not only causes the release of histamines, but also stimulates the formation of mucus in response to sexual activity.(5)

Like zinc, vitamin E is concentrated in the pituitary gland and is essential for the production of sex and adrenal hormones. Acting as an antioxidant, it protects all body organs and glands from destruction by oxygen. It is required for normal brain functioning and reflexes, which are involved in sexual arousal. Vitamin E both directly and indirectly touches every cell of the body, protecting them from aging. It is difficult to obtain the minimum RDA of vitamin E because of the processing and refining of the major portion of our food supply. It helps to include plenty of wheat germ, nuts, seeds, eggs, leafy vegetables, and vegetable oils. If these foods are not a regular part of your diet, you may want to supplement. Most people can take up to 400 IU safely; however, if you have a rheumatic heart or high blood pressure, consult with your doctor before taking any.

Hypothyroidism may be a cause of low sexual desire. A low metabolic rate, suggested by a sluggish thyroid, not only produces fatigue, lethargy, and weight gain, but also may be responsible for decreased sexual interest. Conversely, an overactive thyroid (hyperthyroid), which speeds up the body's basal metabolism, can result in rampant sexuality. People who take thyroid hormones often report an unusually strong interest in sex. A number of nutrients, such as iodine, copper, zinc, and the amino acid tyrosine, are important in activating the thyroid gland in individuals who have low thyroid activity.(6)

Certain foods may inhibit glandular secretion and thus sexual interest: foods like turnips, kale, cabbage, and soybeans, contain an antithyroid substance, and should be avoided by individuals who have decreased thyroid activity. Fasting, although a healthy practice, may inhibit thyroid function. When the body does not get enough calories, it slows down to conserve its energy. Regular fasting may induce a slowed metabolic state and inhibit sexual urges. If you want to increase or maintain your sexual activity, eat regularly.

The adrenal glands are critical to sexual development and drive. If you suffer from adrenal exhaustion, which can be caused by continued external stress (death, divorce, moving, family problems), internal stress (overuse of sugar, fat, coffee, or alcohol), or both, you may not feel very romantic. Finding ways of handling any stress, then, is conducive to a more enjoyable sex life.

Sexual desire and performance can be adversely affected by many things: certain drugs (tranquilizers, muscle relaxants, antidepressants, amphetamines, diuretics, antihypertensives, and hormones, to name a few), alcohol, marijuana, smoking, coffee, overwork, tension, frustration, and depression. The general effects on the body are similar: stress on the adrenal glands and depletion of a wide variety of nutrients.

Recommendations for a Healthy Sex Life

* Find appropriate ways to deal with chronic stress.
* Minimize stress-filled foods: sugar, coffee, alcohol, fried foods, highly processed foods.
* Supplement with major nutrient support: vitamins B, C, and E, and minerals zinc, copper, iodine, magnesium, and calcium.

Chapter 9

———— ❧ ————

Depression

Sometimes I feel like a figment of my own
imagination.

—Lily Tomlin

INTERNALLY OR EXTERNALLY INDUCED

The change of life has long been associated with irritability, nervousness, emotional instability, and depression. If a woman of 50
cries, is irritable, or broods, her feelings are blamed on shifting hormones, just as they were when she was premenstrual or newly pregnant. For some individuals, the phrase "raging hormones" explains
all female complaints. This is a harmful attitude. It may make a
woman feel she has no choice but to give in to her chemical controls. What she *should* do is examine other factors in her life that
may have just as significant an effect on her behavior—family
problems, fear of the change, poor health.

Whether depression and emotional swings during menopause are psychological or biological in origin is still hotly debated
by psychologists, physicians, biochemists, and nutritionists. On
the one hand are those who are convinced that mood swings are
caused by the fluctuating, unstable hormone levels of midlife. On
the other are those who contend that hormones have very little to

do with behavior, that the distraught menopausal woman is one who has succumbed to deep-seated psychological insecurities. A third suggestion, and one heard less often, is that having the "blues" sometimes may be normal at midlife. After all, chemical shifts are not the only changes occurring at that point in the life cycle—family and other relationships, career, and health may likewise be going through transition.

As one who believes that all health—good or ill—is related to the total life experience of an individual, I feel that all these views are viable. We cannot deny that the body is going through a hormonal transition that for some women is abrupt and extreme. Temporary physical and psychological side effects are to be expected. When there is a rapid drop in estrogen and progesterone, or any other hormone for that matter, it is quite possible that psychological reactions will be triggered.

Our emotions are strongly affected by the inner climate of the body, and the more dramatic the change in that climate, the more likely we are to feel uneasy about it. As an illustration, think about how you feel when you are coming down with the flu. You're nauseated, tired, and weak. Everything aches—even your teeth and hair seem to hurt. Not only do you feel physically drained, but your attitude toward the world around you changes. You don't want to talk to people, you're short-tempered, and your outlook in general is anything but positive and uplifting. Your physical condition leads to an emotional state that eases once you are feeling better.

There is another factor that may enter into depression that is often not considered. Emotional problems can be a kind of nonspecific reaction to poor nutrition. A diet lacking in even one vital nutrient can bring about vague mood swings and unexplained depression. If you feel "under the weather" and don't think you are reacting to a stressful situation or a repressed need, look to your eating habits. They may be partially, if not totally, responsible.

Will you be depressed as you go through menopause? It is difficult to predict. But you can start to prepare yourself psychologically by examining honestly how you feel about it. You can also prepare your body physically through diet, exercise, and healthy living.

WOMEN MOST SUSCEPTIBLE TO DEPRESSION

It is a myth that menopause increases the incidence of depression. While menopausal women do seem to complain frequently of feeling "blue and weepy," the proportion in this age group of clinically depressed women requiring help is comparable to any other age group. This suggests either that these women were depressed before the change took place or that they are not experiencing what psychiatrists refer to as "classic" depression.

The sense of feeling unhappy, disoriented, or out of focus is not the true clinical definition of depression. According to Dr. Barbara Edelstein, psychiatric resident at the Eastern Pennsylvania Psychiatric Institute of Living and author of *The Women Doctor's Guide for Women*, "The depressed person is unhappy, discouraged, pessimistic, wiped-out, bored, guilty, disgusted, clumsy, tearful, suicidal, irritable, disinterested, indecisive, unmotivated, sleepless, sexless, helpless, and hopeless."(1) Menopausal women, or any of us for that matter, may experience many of these symptoms at various times in our lives. The difference is that the truly depressed individual experiences a greater number of continuous symptoms to a greater degree.

According to psychotherapists, depression during menopause reaches back into the earlier emotional life of the woman. Traditional psychology teaches that emotional symptoms reflect an underlying conflict the individual is attempting to resolve. If a woman has not come to terms with a particular problem, such as her own identity, her depression could be a continuing issue that flares up at midlife, not a new situation.

A universal characteristic to watch for in a depressed woman is lack of self-esteem. Judging from the higher rates of depression in women compared to men, in both the United States and Europe, women in our culture seem to struggle more than men with role perception and self-identity. Not having a clear awareness of who they are, what they should be doing, and what their purpose in life is creates for women insecurity and doubts about self-worth. This seems to occur especially in married women who do not work outside the home. For example, when a married woman attends a social function, she is often introduced as "Larry's wife," or "Amy's mother." If she has no strong sense of her own identity, going through life being thought of by some only in terms of her relationship to others may make her feel that no one even knows her name.

I would like to share an example from my own experience that typifies the pervasive denial of self among women. A few years ago, I joined a women's study group in the hope of meeting other working and nonworking mothers who were actively involved in managing all the diverse roles women of today are called upon to play. At the first meeting, our group leader asked us each to give our names and then tell what our husbands did for a living—not what *we* did, but what *they* did. My face reddened and I could feel the tremor in my voice even before I spoke. When my turn came, I dutifully gave my name, then explained that it was my intention to get to know more women as individuals. I wanted to know what they did all day, how they felt, and what they thought; and that had nothing to do with their husbands' positions. I think what shocked me most was that I seemed to be the only woman who resented the question.

Studies reveal that most women see themselves in terms of either their physical bodies or their various roles. Psychologist Lillian Rubin found that, when asked to describe themselves, most women started with their physical attributes: "I'm short, tall, blond, fat, pretty, not so pretty anymore, and average."(2) One should not find these responses surprising in a culture where youth and beauty are women's most valued commodities.

These research projects yield more than just interesting psychological accounts. They can be predictive. Women who either are overconcerned with their physical appearance or have defined their role in terms of husbands and children seem to have the most difficulty accepting the change of life.

Role loss is associated with depression, and certain female roles are conducive to increasing the incidence of emotional loss. For example, women who are overprotective of their children are more likely than other women to suffer depression after their children leave home.(3) Excessively devoted mothers—mothers who have sacrificed their lives for their children at the expense of their own interests—are more likely to experience the "empty-nest syndrome" when their children move away.

The emotional life of a woman prior to menopause will determine, at least in part, how she will react to her physiological changes. If she has not defined her identity as a woman in the years prior to menopause, there is strong evidence that menopause may be a difficult emotional transition for her. The best treatment in this case is early recognition and good counseling. Remember, serious depression requires professional care.

Remember also, not all women going through menopause are depressed or sing the blues all day. Some women sail through the change happy, rewarded, and secure—cultural conditioning, hormonal imbalances, and all. Sadja Greenwood, M.D., assistant clinical professor at the University of California Medical Center at San Francisco, feels that women who value themselves in their work (as homemakers or on a job site), women who have interesting jobs, steady incomes, a sense of purpose, and things to do usually report fewer problems with menopause.(4) But to arrive at menopause feeling secure and worthwhile means you have to begin early in life to like and value yourself.

PHYSICAL CAUSES OF DEPRESSION

Biochemical and hormonal factors may induce depression in an otherwise healthy individual. The endocrine and nervous systems are closely linked, and when any hormone, sex related or not, is out of balance, the emotions are affected. For example, during the first several days and even weeks following the birth of a baby, there is an abrupt decline in circulating estrogen, progesterone, and cortisol. This, coupled with the physiological drain of labor, causes many women to experience a significant emotional low known generally as "postpartum depression." Even women who have had an uneventful pregnancy and an easy delivery may experience it. I know I did, and my pregnancy was quite uneventful. No one was more surprised than I to find, after my beautiful daughter was born, that I could feel anything but high on love. I was positive I could care for this tiny infant as well as clean the house, cook meals, wash diapers, and so on. I was certain I would be in control. Almost a week after arriving home, I started crying—for no apparent reason. The guilt I felt about being unhappy when I had everything I wanted made matters worse. If I had been told that these outbursts were related to the physical changes in my body, I might have handled it better. Just knowing something is normal helps immensely.

It has been reported by the Harvard Medical School that there is a difference in various blood hormone levels between depressed and nondepressed people. A sharp drop in hormone levels may lead to significant changes in behavior. Throughout their lives, certain women show greater degrees of hormonal highs and lows. Women who have suffered from premenstrual syndrome (PMS) can testify to the reality of physical and emotional symptoms they experience when their hormones fluctuate. But just as all women don't have PMS, not all women will experience an exaggerated drop in hormones at menopause. By maintaining a healthy body, a woman is less prone to extremes in chemical reactions that can alter normal behavior.

NUTRITION AND THE EMOTIONS

Nutrients—or the lack of them—affect mood, thinking, and behavior. Until recently, physicians who dared to suggest that food might influence emotions were laughed at. Today, however, reputable scientific investigators from noteworthy institutions report on the link, and there is no longer any real controversy. Psychological disturbances are some of the earliest symptoms of nutritional inadequacy.

The fact that hormone levels drop sharply during periods of semistarvation has been reported in the medical literature. Though few of us may fit that description, there is still a great number of individuals who, because of poverty, unsafe dieting, or poor food selection—exist on a substandard diet. Strange as it sounds, women—who are generally the ones who plan, shop for, and prepare meals—seem to be most prone to eating improperly. Government surveys show we barely take in half the RDAs (recommended daily allowances), an already minimum requirement for health.

Biochemically, each individual is unique. Nutritionally, our needs vary as much as the shapes of our bodies. With respect to amino acids alone, direct experimentation has indicated that some people require two, four, or six times as much of a particular substrata of protein as others just to maintain their health.(5) (This fact is most important because of the correlation between depression and amino acids.) The same applies to all the other nutrients.

Dr. Roger Williams, the biochemist who discovered pantothenic acid and who has done extensive original work in the field of vitamin research, discusses the importance of nutrients in the control of mental problems. He says the most important way to improve the environment of the brain cells of a threatened individual is to give them the full nutritional chain of life. The only way the brain cells receive the elements they need is from the individual's diet. When these elements are not provided, a variety of emotional conditions might result.(6) Check and see if any of the symptoms listed below sound familiar to you.

Symptoms and Related Nutrient Deficiencies

* vitamin B-3 (niacin): insomnia, nervousness, irritability, confusion, depression, hallucination
* vitamin B-1 (thiamine): loss of appetite, depression, irritability, memory loss, sensitivity to noise, inability to concentrate
* pantothenic acid: depression, inability to tolerate stress
* vitamin B-12 (cobalamine): difficulty in concentration and remembering, stuporous depression, severe agitation, hallucinations, manic behavior
* potassium: nervousness, irritability, mental disorientation
* magnesium: paranoid psychosis
* calcium: anxiety, neurosis, fatigue, insomnia, tension

The chemical makeup of the brain requires an ample and constant supply of essential nutrients. Vitamins, amino acids, fatty acids, and enzymes are all interrelated, each dependent on the others for absorption and utilization; moreover, a shortage of one vital element can render all the others less effective. Thus, nutritionists urge people to eat a variety of nutrient-dense foods, thereby reducing the possibility of deficiency in any area.

Proper functioning of the brain is more dependent on what we eat than that of any other organ in the body. About ten years ago, Richard Wurtman, M.D., a neuroendocrinologist from MIT, reported the conclusions of his work with neurotransmitters, chemicals through which the brain's nerve cells communicate. He found that the brain's ability to make certain neurotransmitters depended on the amount and type of various nutrients circulating in the blood. Since this discovery, many experiments have demonstrated that by eating certain foods or taking specific vitamins, minerals, and amino acids, an individual can raise the level of brain neurotransmitters and reduce depressive symptoms.

NATURAL "UPPERS"

The natural approach to depression prescribed by nutritionally oriented doctors and psychiatrists includes a combination of vitamins, minerals, and amino acids. (Amino acids are the building blocks of protein; when protein foods are broken down in the body, the end products are amino acids.) Specific amino acids are precursors to the brain neurotransmitters; that is, they are directly involved in the synthesis of such neurotransmitters. The amino acids most commonly recommended for relieving anxiety and depression are L-tryptophan, L- tyrosine, and L-phenylalanine.

Tryptophan is one of the few substances capable of passing through the blood-brain barrier, the sac of membranes that covers the brain tissue and prevents foreign substances from entering. When metabolized in the presence of vitamin B-6, tryptophan is instrumental in synthesizing serotonin, another neurotransmitter that is known to influence mood. In sufficient amounts, this amino acid has an antidepressant effect comparable to that of any major prescription drug. Since the amino acid is natural to the body, the side effects are thought to be considerably fewer and less severe than those associated with antidepressant drugs.

Researchers have found a direct correlation between low estrogen and low tryptophan levels in the blood of depressed menopausal women. Evidence is strong that there may be a chemical relationship in women who have had previous bouts of depression, for example, during the premenstrual period. It would appear that the depression is related to both a hormonal imbalance and a deficiency in tryptophan. At this point, it is difficult to say which comes first, the deficiency or the imbalance. But since supplementary tryptophan relieves the depression, it is a moot point.

Tryptophan is found in a wide variety of foods, including eggs, turkey, soybeans, and dairy products. Women with cyclic imbalances should introduce more of these foods into their diet. To counteract severe depression, however, amounts greater than could be consumed in food alone are needed, and supplementation of L-tryptophan (2–3 gm) is suggested, taken at bedtime or spread throughout the day. The tablets should be ingested with a high carbohydrate meal or snack rather than with protein, because tryptophan can pass readily through the blood-brain barrier only when there is no competition from other amino acids.

L-phenylalanine is another amino acid the body uses to form neurotransmitters. Along with vitamins C and B-6, and pantothenic acid, it is a precursor to norepinephrine and dopamine, chemicals that excite the brain, keeping us alert, ambitious, and self-confident. Certain types of depression respond favorably to L-phenylalanine (1–3 gm) which should be taken on an empty stomach in the morning or at night. Natural sources of phenylalanine include most protein foods, for example, beef, chicken, fish, eggs, almonds, peanuts, and baked beans. Women with hypertension should not take large amounts of phenylalanine.

L-tyrosine is derived from L-phenylalanine, and plays an intermediary role in the synthesis of norepinephrine and dopamine. Reports indicate that tyrosine metabolism may be abnormal in depressed persons.(7) L-tyrosine (2–4 gm) is recommended as an aid in controlling anxiety and depression; it should be taken in the morning, prior to breakfast. Note, however, that people who suffer from migraine headaches and high blood pressure should not take this amino acid in the high doses recommended for depression. Tyrosine breaks down to the chemical tyramine in such foods as aged cheese, beer, wine, yeast, ripe bananas, avocados, and chicken livers. It has been shown that these foods can act as triggers for migraine headaches.

Maintaining a constant level of glucose in the blood is important to one's well-being. The brain and nervous system are especially sensitive to disturbances in blood glucose levels. Even though the central nervous system does not store glucose, it needs more of it than any other part of the body; and the primary part of that system, the brain, is the first to feel the deficiency when the glucose level is low. The brain and nervous system are so hypersensitive to disturbances of body chemistry that a defect in the utilization of sugar can result in an erratic mental state, with a list of symptoms and complaints that read like a compendium on a bottle of snake-oil medicine: dizziness, fainting, headaches, fatigue, muscle pains, cold hands and feet, insomnia, irritability, crying spells, nervous breakdown, excessive worry, depression, illogical fears, suicidal thoughts, crawling sensation, loss of sexual drive—and the list goes on.(8)

Women who consume large amounts of sugar, pastry, white flour, coffee, and alcohol are inviting both mental and physical problems. Despite media reports on the value of a proper diet, many otherwise intelligent women ignore the evidence. It is not easy to give up childhood habits, but it is clear that to build our future health, we must be concerned with good nutrition.

We all experience degrees of sporadic blood-sugar fluctuations at various time in our lives. If you are feeling low and can't explain why, examine your eating habits. Do they include drinking a lot of coffee, tea, and alcohol, and eating inordinate amounts of sugar and processed foods? All of these can be responsible in part for unnatural highs and lows. To stabilize your blood-sugar level, eliminate these stresses from your diet and eat foods high in protein and complex carbohydrates.

The number of meals you eat throughout the day can help as well. Six small meals a day are more conducive to furnishing a slow release of insulin from the pancreas, subsequently allowing for the gradual release of glucose.

I cannot leave this subject without mentioning the benefits of intensive physical exercise in relieving tension and elevating mood. Exercise is now considered more effective in relieving depression than the most commonly used tranquilizers. In 1978, John Grerist, M.D., of the University of Wisconsin, found running to be useful as psychotherapy for depression. Even when the study was over, the once-depressed runners continued to run, finding that when they quit, their depression returned.(9) Running may not be the answer for you, but walking is a good alternative, and there are any number of other forms of exercise you can do. The thing that's important is, if you feel down, do an aerobic exercise, one that gets your heart pumping moderately, for at least 20 minutes, four times a week. It will undoubtedly raise your spirits.

Chapter 10

———— ❧ ————

Women and Stress

Aging results from the sum of all the stresses
to which the body has been exposed during a
lifetime.

—Hans Selye

Stress is a difficult term to define. Hans Selye, considered by many
to be the foremost modern researcher of stress, calls stress a nonspecific (generalized) response of the body to any demand made
upon it. By this definition, whether the stressor is pleasant or painful, the body reacts physically in the same way.

The primary function of the stress reaction is to prepare the
body to act by providing it with energy. Whether the stressor is
positive or negative, real or imagined, physical or emotional, the
body immediately mobilizes all its resources—chemical, physical,
and psychological—for "fight" or "flight." Hormones surge
through the body, the muscles tense, the heart races, the stomach
churns, the hands sweat, and the throat becomes dry. These are
normal reactions to situations in which one is exhilarated, eager,
and ready to act. Selye calls this "eustress" or "good stress," because
it leads to adaptation, accommodation, growth, self-confidence,
and greater resistance to future stresses.

It is important to understand that stress itself is not bad; it is not something to be avoided at all cost. Without it, living would be uneventful and boring. Our goal should be to find a balance between enough stress and too much.

Countless studies show that the average modern life-style is stressful, and many of us have tipped the scales in favor of overload. While emotional strain certainly may be a factor, it is more likely we are suffering from the long-term effects of minor physical stresses. These occur when external forces—heat or cold, overwork, injuries, malnutrition, exposure to drugs and poisons—continually assault the body. For women, certain life passages, such as pregnancy and menopause, combine a high degree of emotional and physical stress, compounding the situation.

Allowing our bodies to function constantly in a state of over-stimulation can be dangerous—so much so, in fact, that stress, or, to be more accurate, distress is now considered the number one social and health problem in the United States and possibly the world. It is one of the major factors correlated with an increase in heart disease, ulcers, hypertension, infections, cancer, and all degenerative diseases. According to the American Academy of Family Physicians, two-thirds of all office visits to family doctors are prompted by stress-related symptoms.(1) Clearly, this is not a subject to be ignored or underrated.

WOMEN'S DILEMMA

Women are now, more than at any time in history, prone to anxiety. As more opportunities open up, our stress levels increase. The multiple roles of mother, homemaker, student, career woman, and concerned citizen require more hours in a day than nature allows.

No matter which roles women assume, it often seems we just can't win. If a woman chooses to remain in the home, she may feel pressured by society to be "productive," to get out in the world and "actualize her potential." If she decides to continue or even start a career after the birth of her children, she's tagged a "working mother," a label that often makes her feel guilt-ridden. Working part-time and spending afternoons with the children isn't always the ideal solution either. When she's at work she feels she should be at home; when she spends her time being mother of the year, she longs for adult stimulation and new challenges. Modern women are torn between difficult choices and perpetual guilt.

It often seems that men don't fully appreciate women's plight—the fact that the woman is the hub around which everything and everyone revolves. When I tried to convey to some male friends my frustration at this situation after a particularly trying day—when, while I was attempting to write at home, my son came in from school with a 101 degree temperature, the water heater broke, a close friend needed a shoulder to cry on, and my daughter's car was totaled—I was reminded, unsympathetically, of the current philosophy that "anyone can do what she wants to do." Even Geraldine Ferraro passes this truism on in her Pepsi commercial. How many times I had read and agreed with that statement— that is, until I tried to put it into practice.

Men are rarely confronted with the multiple distractions facing women both at home and at the office. When children are ill, it is still, unfortunately, almost always the mother who must stay home from work to care for them. Even working at home is usually different for a man than it is for a woman. Dad may ask for and receive quiet while he deals with work, but Mom is less likely to be able to cut herself off from the household's needs while she works. Unless she lives in a truly egalitarian household, the woman is often simply expected to be constantly on call.

Women also often have the double burden of working both outside and inside the home. Although men take part more today than in the past, it is still rare for household chores to be distributed equally. According to Colette Dowling, "Regardless of whether she works full time or has children, or makes more money than her husband does, when it comes to managing the house and taking care of children, the woman always does more."(2) We hear a great deal about new, innovative life-styles, in which fathers assume equal responsibilities at home, but the reality is that these families are still rare. Most home responsibilies still fall to the woman, even if she works full time outside the home.

Sociologist Nora Kinzer informs us that marriage, although a stress-reducing mechanism for men, is a stress-producing one for women.(3) Women need to work to change this balance, clearly, by continuing to demand respect for all their work and by accepting nothing less than equally shared responsibility at home. Obviously, however, we aren't there yet; the home and marriage do add stress to women's lives that they don't add to men's.

STRESS AND SOCIAL CONDITIONING

Stress in women is fostered early in life, as young girls are trained to act and react according to society's or parents' expectations. In my youth, we were taught to be sweet, well-behaved, not too aggressive, and always in control of our behavior. Boys could be boys and get away with it, but for girls to be anything but good was unthinkable. I never considered saying or doing a thing that I thought my parents or church would not condone. The few times I did try my wings convinced me the negative response was not worth the effort. To learn that young girls experience a higher anxiety level than boys because of their struggle to control natural impulses should come as no shock to women of my generation.

Repression of emotion has been shown time and again to cause psychosomatic symptoms. In cultures where venting emotions is encouraged, the incidence of several diseases is reduced. For example, Latins, known for their more exuberant expressiveness, generally have a lower incidence of heart disease and ulcers than do inexpressive Anglo-Saxons.

Another cause of female stress accompanies early childhood training. Fear of success, fear of failure, and the "Cinderella complex" are all terms that describe the modern woman who is unprepared to compete in a formerly "male society." As women realize the opportunities and new career choices available to them, they discover they lack the psychological training needed to achieve these goals. While men are educated and molded for independence, most women are taught to be dependent; thus, when faced with freedom of choice and action, rather than forging ahead, women often retreat. According to Dr. Georgia Witkin-Lanoil, psychiatrist and author of _The Female Stress Syndrome_, "It's not uncommon for women to feel a mixture of the fear of failure and the need for achievement."(4) The head-on collision between the two is what she titles the "female stress syndrome."

Necessary to overcoming any fear is recognizing exactly what it is we fear. In his book *Fear of Success*, David Ward Tresmer cites the work of Dr. Matina Horner, possibly the foremost researcher in this field. Dr. Horner writes that the main fear women have about doing well professionally is that they may jeopardize their relations with men.(5) More than realizing their own dreams, many women want a close relationship with a man, so much so that they will sabotage their own success. Many women remain ambivalent about which role they want for fear of losing what they already have. They are not willing to commit themselves totally because the consequences, whatever they may be, are unknown. Not having experienced risk-taking situations, women tend to move forward hesitantly, to hold back, hedging their bets, trying to achieve success in a competitive world without giving up old-fashioned, "feminine" ways.(6)

Many women are torn between what we were brought up to believe and what we now recognize we can achieve. The internal role conflicts lead to stress from which women had previously been protected. The fact that women now experience typical male "stress" diseases like heart disease and hypertension is proof of increased anxiety. To protect our future health, it is imperative that we find ways to cope with what we have been taught and what we now want our lives to be.

REACTING TO STRESS

The manner in which one responds to stress is actually more important than the stress-producing situation. Consequently, much of the research concerning the prevention of harmful effects of stress looks into coping mechanisms. Psychologists believe that the first step paramount to coping successfully is the sense of being in control of one's life. Many mothers fall naturally into the category of people who feel they have little control over their lives, because their schedules are dependent on those of all the other family members, and their personal desires or work routines are sacrificed to the needs of their families.

Recognizing that inconveniences and distractions are inevitable is necessary in maintaining your feeling of being in control. It is natural to become frustrated and angry when unexpected events disrupt your plans, but it is much healthier in the long run to accept what has happened and adapt. Robert Eliot, a cardiologist from the University of Nebraska, has some great rules for coping with stress:

> Rule No. 1 is, don't sweat the small stuff.
> Rule No. 2 is, it's all small stuff.
> And, if you can't fight and you can't flee, flow.

STRESS VERSUS DISTRESS

There is a difference between productive stress (eustress) and its counterpart, distress. While eustress is exhilarating, distress is injurious (see Figure 6). The normal adaptive stress cycle occurs when the source of the stress is generally short term and identifiable. Upon overcoming or adapting to the challenge, the individual rests, thereby reestablishing normal body functioning before the next stressor arises. A resting stage is most important to the normal adaptive cycle. When the body recovers completely, it can prepare for the next stressor. The more intense the stressor, the longer the period of deep rest and recovery must be.

Should the stress be long-term, ambiguous, and undefined, or if several stressful situations exist simultaneously, the individual will not have a chance to rest completely or return to a normal level. When the body remains in a heightened state of arousal for weeks, months, or even years, the resting stage deteriorates into exhaustion. Organ systems collapse, the adrenal glands shrink, hormones are depleted, the immune system becomes inefficient, and eventually the ability to adapt is lost. At the very least, the individual experiences physical and emotional manifestations, such as sweaty palms, nervousness, fidgeting, tight lips, shaking, squinting eyes, teeth gritting, biting nails, back pain, insomnia, inability to relax, compulsive eating, PMS, pounding heart, nervous tics, indigestion, dry mouth and throat, headaches, and hypertension. At the extreme, more serious stage of exhaustion, there may be severe damage to body tissues, premature aging, impairment of the immune system, and even death.

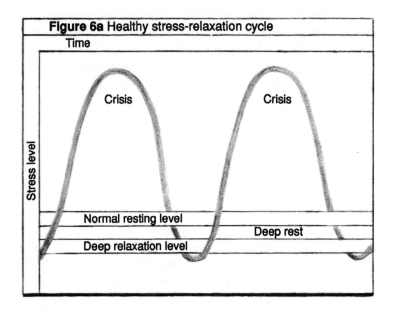

Figure 6a Healthy stress-relaxation cycle

Time

Stress level

Crisis

Crisis

Normal resting level

Deep rest

Deep relaxation level

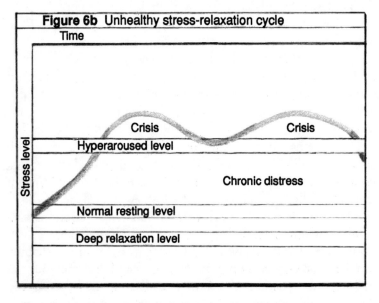

Figure 6b Unhealthy stress-relaxation cycle

Time

Stress level

Crisis

Crisis

Hyperaroused level

Chronic distress

Normal resting level

Deep relaxation level

Distress can be the result of one traumatic incident or several long-term conditions. A person may be totally overwhelmed by the thought of living alone after 30 years of marriage, by a death in the family, or the loss of a home by fire, for example. Likewise, the compound effects of one change after another—a new house, new job, and new mate all at one, for instance—may equally shock the system.

In an attempt to measure the impact of common "life changes," psychiatrist Thomas Holmes and psychologist Richard Rahe worked out a numerical scale of values for the significant events of life. As might be expected, at the top of the list is the death of a spouse, followed by divorce, marital separation, retirement, and pregnancy. Interestingly, there is no category for menopause on the Holmes/Rahe Scale, even though it is considered a significant life change. However, if you add up typical changes that often coincidentally occur at menopause, such as change in work, children leaving home, wife starting to work, change in living conditions, revision of personal habits, change in health of family member, and change in eating and sleeping habits, you could easily total 300 points, the number researchers feel would increase your risk of becoming seriously ill or vulnerable to depression. These scores are by no means precise predictors of who will get sick; they merely confirm the correlations among life changes, stress, and physical and emotional health.

Psychologist Richard Lazarus, Ph.D., and his colleagues at the University of California at Berkeley found that "daily hassles may have a greater effect on our moods and our health than the major misfortunes of life."(7) Unfortunately, we are not always cognizant of the seemingly insignificant aggravations that over the years wear down our bodies: commuting daily in heavy traffic, feeling that there is not enough time for the family or work, friction with a coworker or neighbor. Even something as innocuous as constant noise can, over a period of time, exhaust our stress response. Researchers have tested people living near the Los Angeles International Airport and have found a higher rate of hypertension, heart disease, and suicide among them than in residents of quieter areas.

Further, air and water pollution, smoking, and diets that include excessive alcohol, sugar, and junk foods all evoke the stress response. Many people don't realize how much we are bombarded daily by stress-provoking stimulants. Certainly it is not possible to control each and every environmental aggravation, but you can use the known stressors discussed above as a guide for improving your own surroundings. How well you cope with the physical and psychological symptoms of menopause may depend on the reduction of distress in your life all the years before.

NUTRITIONAL SUPPORT FOR COPING WITH STRESS

How we cope with everyday stress, whether internal or external, depends directly on the overall condition of our organs and glands. Obviously, some people inherit stronger sets of glands and can handle far more abuse than others. But even in healthy individuals, age generally decreases the ability to adapt. The older we get, the more concerned we need to be with the unnecessary stressors in our lives.

Stress can be a constant drain on the adrenal glands, and since these glands play a major supportive role during and after menopause, it is imperative that we pamper them throughout our early years. The first step for ensuring healthy glands is to stay close to nature in the food we eat. If you have overworked your glands throughout your younger years, if you are prone to hypoglycemia, PMS, or emotional problems, you may need to counteract the harmful effects of a poor diet with additional nutrients.

The body's response to most stress is to manufacture more adrenalin. An increase in adrenalin speeds up the metabolization of protein, fats, and carbohydrates, producing the surge of energy we characteristically notice. A side effect of the increased metabolization, however, is a loss of body protein, potassium, and phosphorus and a decreased storage of calcium. Many of the disorders blamed on stress are a consequence of nutrient deficiencies caused by the increased metabolic rate during the period of stress. For example, vitamin C, which is concentrated in the adrenal glands and organs of high metabolic activity, is utilized by the adrenals during anxiety-producing situations. Any type of stress, severe or prolonged, will cause a depletion of vitamin C in the tissues. Being deficient in vitamin C is itself a threat to the system.

All of the B vitamins support adrenal functioning. Dr. Michael Jefferson, a British neurologist, has found B-vitamin deficiencies to be responsible for many of the complaints associated with middle age because of their invaluable effect not only on the adrenals but also on the nervous system.(8) B vitamins function as enzymes in carbohydrate metabolism, which is the keystone for proper functioning of nerve cells.

The adrenal glands cannot function without potassium. Even though potassium is found in a wide variety of fresh fruits and vegetables, it can easily be depleted, rendering the body deficient and unprotected. You may be compromising your potassium balance if you diet frequently, sweat excessively, take diuretics or steroids, or eat too much salt. If you absolutely cannot stand the thought of giving away your salt shaker, try some of the new salt substitutes that are high in potassium chloride. The other problems speak for themselves.

Individuals who are continually subjected to stress will require additional fortification. Supplementing with B vitamins and vitamin C provides only a handful of the necessary nutrients significant to maintaining healthy adrenal glands. You need the full spectrum. Many companies now have come out with stress formulas that include these basic nutrients, as well as other nutritional supports for healthy glands. A multiple vitamin/mineral supplement can likewise be an additional reinforcement for temporary periods of distress.

LIFE-STYLE FACTORS

This may sound strange, but stress on one system helps to relax another. That is why exercise is so beneficial in relieving anxiety and nonspecific stress responses. For short-term or emergency stress, exercise can be both physical and emotional catharsis. As pain-relieving hormones pour throughout the system, one experiences feelings of well-being and contentment. Once the stress response is in full gear and the adrenalin is forcing fatty acids and sugar into the blood, we need exercise to normalize and reestablish hormonal balance. If it is not controlled through physical exercise, which is often the case, it may be channeled inward to one of the organ systems, such as the digestive, circulatory, or nervous system. You probably already know the outcome of overactive stress hormones: fatigue, insomnia, backache, hypertension, ulcers, asthma, allergic reactions, and atherosclerosis. It has been proven time and again that a person who is in good physical condition is generally better prepared to withstand the ill effects of stress.

In the management of stress, learning to relax is extremely important. Quick tips written up in popular periodicals are useful: take a hot bath, listen to classical music, go for a long walk, breathe deeply, have a massage, read a good novel, visit friends, or go shopping. Get away, at least temporarily, from the stressful situation or environment, and do something you enjoy. Integrate this into your life-style. Sometimes, however, more energy must be directed toward creating a deeper form of mental relaxation in order to quiet the stress response. For centuries, meditation, prayer, and yoga have shown that it is possible to induce states of deep physical relaxation through definite, well-established techniques. Recent scientific evidence has confirmed that such practices are, in fact, most beneficial in relieving the tension of everyday living and can possibly prevent stress-related diseases.

Herbert Benson, M.D., of the Harvard Medical School, has worked with relaxation techniques for more than ten years. He has clearly defined and measured the physiological effects of these various mental techniques and has found that the biochemical changes that occur through relaxation can help the body to counteract the "fight-or-flight" response and bring about the deep relaxation necessary to stress recovery. Dr. Benson believes this temporary slowdown of body processes repeated twice a day is responsible for the improved health of his subjects. Numerous researchers have confirmed similar changes in the body:

* oxygen consumption decreased
* heart rate decreased
* respiratory rate decreased
* blood pressure rate decreased
* muscle tension decreased

All the meditative practices of both the Eastern and Western cultural traditions have been grounded in four basic components that are needed to evoke what Dr. Benson refers to as the "relaxation response": (i) a quiet environment; (ii) a mental device, such as a word or phrase to be repeated in a specific fashion; (iii) the adoption of a passive attitude, which is perhaps the most important element; and (iv) a comfortable position. Practicing this relaxation technique for 10 to 20 minutes once or twice daily should markedly enhance your sense of well-being.

Chapter 11

— ❧ —

Weight Control

Obesity is but a symptom. It means that something is wrong. When you eat the food your
body is constructed to eat, you will lose the
symptom.

—Lendon Smith, M.D.

MIDDLE-AGE SPREAD

If we're not on guard, middle-age spread can creep up on any of us
past 30. After this age, the body starts to change; muscle tissue
decreases and the body's basal metabolic rate (BMR) slows down.
The BMR reflects the energy required to support basic functions
of life (heart rate, breathing, brain and neural activity, and organ
function). As the BMR goes down, our ability to burn calories is
reduced, therefore, we cannot eat the same amount of calories as
we get older and still maintain our same weight (see Figure 7). In
order to keep the same weight we must ingest fewer calories, become more physically active, or both.

Obviously, monitoring your weight throughout your life is far
better than discovering you have a serious problem at menopause.
Menopause brings enough changes and stresses to contend with;
you don't need to compound the situation by having to lose weight

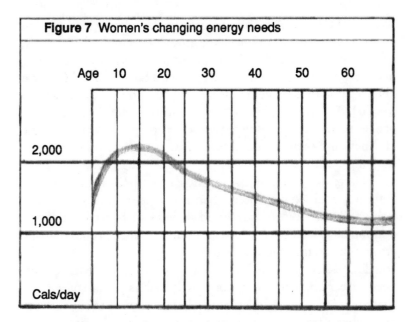

Figure 7 Women's changing energy needs

as well. The best method I know to maintain your figure is to vow never to buy a size larger in clothes. Fitness expert Sheila Cluff suggests always keeping one pair of tight pants and never growing out of them. As soon as they feel too snug or you find you are tugging at the zipper, take action; reduce food intake or increase physical activity. You may not even be eating more than the amount that has always been normal for you, but your body is telling you the time has come for adjustments.

You don't need a scale to tell you it's time to trim off a few inches. In fact, I suggest you throw it out. A scale is not an accurate indicator of fat loss. It doesn't tell you how your body should look or how healthy you are. Worst of all, it is a constant source of anxiety and guilt. When you step on the scale after starving yourself for three days and it reads two pounds higher than you expect, you immediately get depressed. On the other hand, if it reads two pounds lower, the rush of achievement can send you straight to the nearest bakery. It's a no-win situation. Use the "pants approach." It's more reliable and less likely to generate that conditioned punishment/reward response.

When you get older, is it really all that important to keep

your weight down? After all, the dreams of modeling high-fashion dresses on the cover of *Vogue* have long since vanished. Certainly, a few additional pounds won't harm most women. However, being overweight to the point of obesity can be a health hazard (clinical obesity is defined as being 20 percent over one's recommended weight). According to the National Institutes of Health, any level of obesity should be considered a risk factor—just as serious a cause of illness and premature death, in fact, as high blood pressure or smoking.

Carrying around extra weight can be unhealthy, and it is definitely an inconvenience when it comes to buying the latest fashion. But what if you have tried all of the diets in the bookstore and you have lost, gained, lost, and gained so many times that you are convinced it is impossible for you ever to maintain the weight you desire? Are you hopeless? No, you definitely are not. You just need to learn how the body works, what habits you are promoting that prevent your weight loss, and what you can do to change your body chemistry from fat storing to fat burning. Losing fat is a biochemical process, and there is a correct way of encouraging this process to act in your favor. You *can* lose unwanted pounds and keep them off for life.

MOST DIETS DON'T WORK

Most diets do not work in terms of keeping excess weight off permanently. Sure, you lose pounds, but the loss is temporary; once you resume your normal eating habits, the fat finds its way back to its favorite places. There are two primary reasons diets fail. The first is, most diets are foreign to the way people are used to eating. Many people follow strict low-calorie menus or use special drinks until the scale shows the right numbers, then it's back to potato chips, double cheeseburgers, and hot-fudge sundaes. A diet must change your approach to eating in the long term, or you will not maintain any weight loss.

The second reason diets fail is that very low caloric intake changes the body metabolism to promote weight gain. When you go on a crash diet of, say, nothing but grapefruit and peanuts, you actually encourage the storage of fat. As caloric intake is greatly reduced, the body does everything it can to conserve energy. It lowers the metabolic rate to protect you from starving. The more quickly pounds dissolve (especially if it is more than two pounds a week), the more intensely the body hoards its fat. You may lose weight initially, but the pounds you are burning are from your lean muscle tissue rather than from fat stores. Biochemically, your body changes. When muscle mass is decreased, the basal metabolic rate slows down. This means you are burning fewer calories than you did before you started dieting. So, when you return to "normal" eating, it is even easier to gain weight than it was before.

Crash diets are counterproductive in more ways than one. Reducing calories to bare minimum levels usually means reducing nutrient stores as well. When the system is depleted of its vitamins and minerals, it triggers the appetite mechanism in the brain to replenish its supply. Result? You are starved. Bingeing and compulsive eating are common among frequent dieters.

When women "blitz," they tend to cut fat entirely out of their plans. This, too, is both unhealthy and ineffective. A good rule is never to follow any diet that eliminates an entire food group—fat, carbohydrates, or proteins. All are needed. If you eliminate fats completely, you may soon develop dry and brittle hair, dandruff, swelling in the hands and feet, acne, and loss of sex drive. Ironically, one essential fatty acid, linoleic acid, helps burn fat. So, restrict your intake of fats but don't eliminate them entirely.

Frequent and drastic dieting is an emotional nightmare for many women. A study was made at the Mayo Clinic with a group of young, healthy women, women who had no reason to lose weight, but volunteered for the sake of science. They lived together in the clinic, ate a restricted diet, and were tested continually for side effects. "Before three months had passed, the women's personalities underwent startling changes. They began to quarrel endlessly with one another, experienced unprovoked feelings of anxiety, persecution, and hostility. Some suffered nightmares; others felt extreme panic at times. . . . Their memories became faulty; they were clumsy and had trouble paying attention to assigned tasks."(1) Remember, before the experiment these women were emotionally healthy and not overweight; they were exposed to only one reducing diet, yet they suffered great anxiety.

Dieting is a stress to the body both physically and emotionally. Individuals who have experimented with one diet after another are forced to deal not only with the normal anxiety of dieting but the psychological repercussions of failing, the feelings of guilt, frustration, and ego deflation. Crash diets, fad diets, and minimum-calorie diets are unhealthy for the mind as well as for the body. Their benefits are temporary at best; their side effects are multiple and potentially dangerous. So what's the solution?

THE PROPER ATTITUDE

The place to begin is with basic attitude toward dieting and good health. We live in a society where we have been conditioned to expect instant results. Simple over-the-counter remedies are available for almost every ache or pain; for a headache or a fever, we simply take a pill. If we're overweight, we look for a magic pill to swallow at bedtime that will dissolve all our unwanted bulges as we slumber. Clearly, the dollars we shell out for such overnight cures would be far better spent on whole, nutritious foods and a pair of walking shoes. Whether you want good health or a slim body, the only way to achieve it is through a constant daily routine of good health habits.

You cannot keep pounds off your body permanently until you realize that the foods you eat on your "weight-loss program" must be similar to the foods you will choose for the rest of your life. A diet is not temporary, it's a way of living that you maintain on a regular basis. The emphasis needs to be taken away from short-term deprivation and placed on the long-term changes.

It is necessary to retrain your mind to focus on "eating for life" those foods that cause you to feel good, alive, energetic, young, and positive about yourself. It is an attitude concerned with "what is good for my wonderful body" rather than "what I have to give up so I can lose ten pounds by Saturday night."

All eating behaviors are learned; therefore, unhealthy habits can be unlearned and replaced with more positive behaviors. In reality, this sounds easier than it is. Destructive thoughts and practices concerning food and eating have become so much a part of our lives, we don't even realize they exist. Before making changes, we need to take some time to discover some of our inappropriate attitudes and behaviors about food. We need to examine why we eat or overeat, when we eat, and what we may be doing in terms of our eating that may be preventing us from losing weight.

Some examples of unhealthy attitudes you may have concerning food include these:

* I must eat everything on my plate. (*What if you're full?*)
* It's wasteful to throw food away. (*What if you really don't like it?*)
* I can't imagine myself thin. (*Keep practicing.*)
* I'm just a fast eater. (*You will enjoy your food longer if you savor each bite.*)
* I won't enjoy eating if I have to change. (*Try it first and then see.*)
* I've never kept my weight off. I'm meant to be fat. (*There are reasons the weight has returned after dieting. Find out what they are.*)

All of these statements are counterproductive to permanent weight loss. If you believe any of these, you need to rebuild new, more positive thought patterns.

EVALUATING YOUR EATING HABITS

People eat for countless reasons that have nothing to do with hunger. We eat to be sociable, to be accepted. We eat out of boredom, frustration, anger, acceptance, and habit—most of all, habit. And often we aren't even conscious of what we're doing. When you were pouring out your soul to the neighbor next door, how many cups of coffee and halves of doughnuts did you devour? As you wait for the banquet dinner to be served, do you keep track of the rolls and butter or the glasses of wine poured? Situations like this are common, especially among overweight women.

Research has found that many overweight women have completely lost the sensation of hunger. They cannot differentiate it from other feelings. Eating has become their universal response to all emotion. Therefore, no matter what or how they feel, they seek to satisfy themselves with food. One of the first aspects of food control is to determine when you are eating out of genuine hunger and when you are eating to fulfill a secondary need.

I find charting eating habits to be the best way to record caloric intake, as well as to track faulty eating patterns. Using the following chart, write down—and be specific—everything you eat and drink for three weeks. This extended time frame is necessary to cover a wide variety of occasions and experiences—your period, social situations, family get-togethers, and so on that can affect your eating habits. You will be amazed by the different kinds of foods you select when you are alone or with relatives, at parties, and during your period.

In addition to the *kinds* and *amounts* of food you eat, record the *time* that you ate and what you were doing (watching TV, reading the paper, getting dressed, feeding the baby). Very often when we are involved in another activity besides eating, we forget that we have eaten, and repeat the process shortly thereafter. Finally, record how you *felt* while you were eating—relaxed, bored, angry, upset, nervous, or nothing in particular? Were you really hungry for food, or did you have some other need to meet?

By the time you complete the three weeks, you will know a great deal more about your day-to-day eating patterns. How much of your diet is made up of nutrient-rich foods and how much is junk food? To emphasize how many nonfoods you consume, highlight the foods high in fat with a red pen; do the same with sugar-rich foods and a yellow pen. Examples of fatty foods include sausage, bacon, steaks, TV dinners, butter, cream, mayonnaise, salad dressings, margarine, pies, cakes, cookies, and anything fried. Sugary foods may be the same as high-fat foods—they are frequently found together. Some of these are doughnuts, ice cream, soda pop, pastries, and desserts. Most people are shocked to see how great a proportion of their daily diets is made up of these foods.

Just as important as what, where, and why you eat is how often you eat. Do you go all day without eating anything and then gorge before going to bed? Barbara Edelstein, M.D., author of *The Woman Doctor's Diet for Women*, believes strongly in balanced meals throughout the day. It is her opinion that the female body

Daily Eating Behavior Diary

Time	Food (Type and Quantity)	Activity While Eating	Location	Thoughts and Feelings	Action Plan
6:00 am	juice	getting dressed	bedroom	no time to eat	wake up 15 minutes earlier tomorrow
10:00 am	2 doughnuts coffee	talking to coworker	lunchroom	low energy, needed a pickup ate too fast	(1) eat one doughnut more slowly (2) get muffin or bring bagel
1:00 pm	tostada with sour cream and quacamole pop cheesecake	read newspaper and ate alone	restaurant	eat something healthy need dessert	(1) take sour cream off food and just taste guacamole (2) don't eat shell (3) take mints to satisfy sweet tooth
3:00 pm	diet pop	working	work	thirsty just want something	water is a better choice
8:00 pm	3-4 glasses white wine chips vegetables and dip salad with dressing 2 rolls with butter chicken in cream sauce steamed vegetables rice chocolate cake coffee with cream	dinner meeting	hotel banquet room	these people make me nervous look busy, eat I paid for this food so I'm going to eat it	(1) wine spritzer (2) sip wine slowly (3) eat vegetables without dip (4) just taste roll and butter (5) scrape most of cream sauce off food (6) just taste cake (7) take coffee black

cannot metabolize more than a certain number of calories per meal; if this amount is exceeded, the excess will be stored as fat.(2) While the idea of eating several meals may sound counterproductive to losing weight, it really is not. The following study cited by Dr. Edelstein illustrates this important point.

Volunteers were divided into four groups, and given a basic calorie-restricted diet. The first group balanced 1,000 calories among three meals throughout the day and lost two pounds per week. The second group ate no breakfast, had 250 calories for lunch and 500 calories for dinner. They, too, lost two pounds, even though they consumed only 750 calories. The third group ate only 500 calories—all for dinner—and also lost the same amount. Personally, I would rather have the freedom to eat twice as much if the weight loss is the same. The fourth group consumed 1,000 calories, all at dinner, and lost less weight than any of the others. So it does appear that small but frequent meals spread throughout the day are more conducive to weight loss and health.

If you have a weight challenge, it is vital to examine the whats, whens, and whys of your eating behavior. Until you know what you are doing, you cannot make informed choices and changes. Once you have determined what you are eating or doing that promotes weight gain, you must develop a plan for change. Start with the types and quantities of foods you find on your chart. What foods can you cut out completely, or at least cut down on? Don't choose something you dearly love. Make it easy on yourself, and go for those things that you indiscriminately put in your mouth. For example, could you leave out second helpings, the fifth and sixth cookies, or the snacks you grab while making dinner? Next, consider how you might substitute lower-calorie foods for things you regularly eat. For instance, try frozen yogurt for ice cream, low-calorie dressing for regular, nonfat milk for whole, bagels for danish. If you can't tell the difference or if you still feel satisfied with the substitutions, why not eat less? Making these few changes in your diet may be enough to obtain the weight you desire.

Remember to start slowly. Changing habits permanently is never easy, so allow yourself to adjust gradually over a month or two-month period. Look at your chart. Which of your unhealthy habits can you tackle first? Choose one that won't cause you too much stress, yet will give you a feeling of accomplishment. When you've made one successful change, move on to another.

There are many tips for fostering healthy eating and weight loss. I suggest that, as you consciously plan new strategies, you use the following list for new ideas.

Creating New Eating Habits

* Eat at least three meals a day. Skipping meals promotes the starvation response and promotes the storage of fat.

* Get into the habit of talking to your food. Before eating, ask it, "Do I want you? Do I need you? Are you going to make me feel good or bad when I'm finished?"

* Eat without distractions: no TV, radio, newspaper, or book. Concentrate only on the food.

* Create a relaxing, positive environment.

* Eat slowly, enjoying the aroma, color, taste, and texture of the food.

* Eat sitting down. You will be less likely to forget what's gone into your mouth.

* Practice leaving a few bites on your plate at each meal. This teaches self-control.

* Eat with friends, family, or co-workers. Overweight people often feel they must prove to others they are trying to lose weight, so they limit their selections to lettuce and cottage cheese in public, only to binge in solitude. Eat your favorite foods with your friends. Chances are you won't feel the need to overeat later.

* Make a list of activities that make you feel good: reading a novel, watching soap operas, going to the movies, getting a facial, going shopping.

* If you *must* have a hot-fudge sundae, go ahead. But don't chastise yourself. There is no place for guilt in weight management. Besides, no one's perfect.

EXERCISE IS A MUST

Dieting without exercise has a serious drawback; you may lose as much lean muscle tissue as you do fat. Low caloric intake triggers a body process called gluconeogenesis (the process of converting protein to glucose). This process actually breaks down muscle tissue to be used for energy in place of sugar. Because of this action, a person who loses 20 pounds of weight from dieting alone will often lose as much as 10 pounds of muscle. While this looks good on the scales, the muscle loss lowers metabolic rate and therefore increases the chances of regaining the weight.

Exercise, on the other hand, builds muscle mass, thereby raising the BMR. Even moderate exercise increases the metabolic rate three to eight times. And there is a residual effect of regular exercise that keeps the metabolic rate higher than normal for several hours afterward, allowing you to burn more calories even when you are not working at it.

Exercise can change the body's chemistry. When biopsies from endurance athletes were compared to those of untrained college students, it was found that the athletes had a greater number of fat-burning enzymes. However, after the untrained person engaged in endurance exercise for several months, those enzymes increased in number. Apparently, in people who exercise regularly, the body "revs up" the metabolic system to burn fat more efficiently while protecting the muscle tissue.

Exercise affects many hormonal systems in the body. It increases the responsiveness of cells to insulin so that the insulin does not cause increased fat storage. Stress-related hormones like adrenalin and cortisol are metabolized by exercise, which decreases their effect on fat storage. Endorphins, chemicals secreted in the brain as a result of endurance exercise, cause a feeling of well-being and alleviate depression. Many chemical reactions occur from continued exercise that change the body from one that likes to store fat to one that likes to burn fat.

There's no alternative to a sound exercise program for burning fat. It must be included in any weight-loss program.

TAPPING INTO YOUR MIND POWER— INTERVIEW: BOBBE SOMMER, PH.D.

In order to provide the most up-to-date practical advice on weight management, I interviewed Bobbe Sommer, Ph.D., licensed psychotherapist in San Clemente, California, author, and weight management expert. In her book, *Not Another Diet Book* (see the "Resources" section at the end of this book), Dr. Sommer explains how instrumental the brain can be in obtaining, maintaining, and sustaining ideal weight.

Linda: I talk to many women who are perpetually on a diet, yet they either don't lose weight or they lose it temporarily and regain it shortly thereafter. In your experience, why is this true? Why don't diets work?

Bobbe: The reasons they don't work psychologically is because they are deprivation-reward systems. Whenever we deprive ourselves of something we want, at some point we feel we need to be rewarded. "I've punished myself for so long and I've been so good, now I deserve to go out and have a hot-fudge sundae." This is how most people think. They consider eating good food in a regimented way as deprivation. We've been brought up on candy and sweets and popcorn and all that junk, so when we don't have it we feel we're lacking something. Then the media comes along and reinforces that feeling by insisting, "Wouldn't you love to have a taco? Don't you want to feel great today? Sure, you deserve a break. Treat yourself to whatever."

Most of the people I see are fighting a losing battle. Of course they lose weight, but for how long? The premise of a majority of women is that they are going to diet down for the cocktail party and once that is over, it's business as usual. By definition a diet is something people go on for a given length of time until they can go back to their "normal" life and their faulty problem-solving methods of food abuse. That doesn't work. Weight management must be a lifetime commitment to be effective.

Linda: You mentioned faulty thinking patterns. How do we develop them?

Bobbe: Most of us pick up faulty beliefs from early-childhood events. Some of the experiences were overt, obvious statements which were made to us verbally. Other messages were not so obvious. Perhaps they were directed to us in a nonverbal manner but still carried the same power as the overt, verbal messages.

Linda: Would you elaborate on these not-so-obvious childhood tapes?

Bobbe: Sure. Much of what we believe to be true may actually be a lie. When you and I were young and experienced actual pangs of hunger, we knew if we cried, we would get prompt relief. Someone would soon come along and shove a warm bottle in our mouth and we were soon sated. We were also cuddled and held close to Mommy. Let's examine this close association with food and security and/or love only 30 years later. We may still be responding to this associational behavior. Now we sometimes think we are hungry because we experience an emotion that may indeed trigger feelings of uneasiness in our abdominal area. We reach for our famous tension reducer because it worked so well 30 years ago. We have misconstrued the feelings of anxiety in the "pit of our stomachs" to be those of hunger pangs and have acted inappropriately.

This leads to a theory I've come to call "being fat is the result of faulty problem solving." It occurs to me that many of us have attempted to solve our current problems with old, formerly appropriate methods. I feel we are caught in this syndrome until we are able to identify what emotions we are actually experiencing. Once we bring this emotion to awareness level, then we can choose to take action. Once we learn to make our emotions conscious, then we are freed of the time-old compulsion to eat every time we have a pang in the tummy. These feelings of discomfort must be separated from the real feelings of physical hunger. We must learn to distinguish true physical hunger from what I've come to call "head hunger." These head hungers are memory traces of how great it was to be fed, held, loved, burped, and taken care of all in one shot.

Linda: Are you saying that weight problems are unconscious?

Bobbe: That's right. I know it is often difficult for us to truly accept that our weight problem is unconscious, that our thought patterns dictate body weight. But the body will manifest, that is, bring into being, those thoughts that we hold in our minds, whether these thoughts are within our conscious or unconscious mind. The body merely carries out the orders of these thoughts. Our bodies reflect what we think about food and our need or supposed need, for food. Everything in this whole universe proceeds from thought to action to form. For example, I have a thought, "I'm hungry." I take action; I eat. Then I experience form; my body weight changes. When life proceeds in a nice, orderly, uncomplicated manner with all systems "go," this process is wonderful. The Catch-22 comes when I complicate things in such a way as, "I think I'm hungry when in reality I'm bored." This faulty thinking starts the chain process and then I eat as a direct consequence of my faulty thinking pattern. Perhaps I've chained my emotions to food. Many of us do just that. We've learned to substitute the thought of food to reduce tensions that come from our emotions.

Linda: It seems, then, that in order to control weight, we must be made aware of our behavioral patterns. Is this where you're heading?

Bobbe: Yes. The basic aim of any weight-management program is to make what was formerly subconscious, conscious. Only then can you make the decision if you want that cookie. If you decide you do, then go for it and don't feel guilty. But don't eat by default. People actually put themselves into situations where they can go into unconsciousness. They don't even know what they have eaten. A classic example is eating in front of the TV.

Linda: What are some practical suggestions that you can give us?

Bobbe: It's important to be aware of your eating cues. There are place cues, activity cues, and time cues. Overweight people are much more susceptible to external or environmental cues. The media know this and they are geared for it. "Aren't you hungry?" asks a famous advertiser. As you bring your temptations into conscious awareness, you begin to take control of the behaviors and you begin to change them. A daily journal is a useful tool. Write down every morsel that passes your lips and the time you eat. Look for patterns. It's amazing how often we will put the food down if we have to record it. Write down when you ate out of "head hunger." Write down emotional conflict when you are tempted to eat. Do all you can do to raise your conscious awareness. We can't change a behavior until we are aware of the feeling behind it. I like to tell people to "have a plan in hand." Know what you're going to eat for one day at a time. If you blow it, know what you will do the next day to compensate. I always eat more on the weekends, so on Monday I jog farther. It's a constant give-and-take. You have to continually find out the balance that is right for you.

Linda: As a psychologist, do you find that some women require intensive counseling to uncover faulty eating patterns?

Bobbe: Well, it depends. For those women who are obese, yes, many do require individual counseling because there is usually pathology involved. It's more than just the food they consume. There is neurotic behavior that compels them to consume two or three gallons of ice cream at one sitting. Now, when you're dealing with the average person who just wants to lose ten pounds, intensive psychological counseling is not necessary. Some women just aren't aware of what they have to do to take and keep those pounds off. Dieting is not enough, though. They need to exercise and change some of their faulty eating habits as well.

Linda: Do you find the reinforcement of a small group to be more conducive to lasting changes than trying to do it alone?

Bobbe: At times it's almost mandatory. I have been involved in many small- and large-group programs and know how motivating they can be. Psychotherapists even have found—this came when Alcoholics Anonymous was formed—that sometimes self-help groups are every bit as valuable as a therapist. I do think, though, that you need a professional to guide the group, to give it direction, and to keep it to one purpose. It's the whole thing of, "So, Linda, how did you do this week? Not great? Well, what do you want to do differently next week? What have you written down?" It keeps people accountable.

Linda: In your book, *Not Another Diet Book*, you talk about the differences in the right and left brain and how the right brain can help you lose weight. Can you explain the principle for me?

Bobbe: I would love to. Theoretically, most people—93 percent of the population—are left-brain, lateral-dominant, which means that the left brain is the part in which they store verbalization ability, linguistic skills, reading, writing, arithmetic, logical reasoning, planning, goal-setting—that kind of thing. For 7 percent of the population, it is reversed and the right side is dominant. We know that people who have strokes in which their left brain is affected become aphasic. On the other hand, if the stroke affects the right side of the brain, this rarely occurs. The right brain is what we call the holistic, pictorial side. It seems to see the whole picture. Only the right side of your brain can recognize another human face. The left side says, "There are two eyes, a nose, an ear, and another ear; OK, that's a face." But it doesn't put it together. The right brain says, "Oh, that's Linda." The right brain picks up subtleties, innuendoes, and the emotional things that the left brain cannot. It just gets the facts, that's it. Theoretically, in a well-balanced brain the left side is feeding the right side factual information and the right side interprets it. There's a constant feedback between them. The vehicle by which the left brain makes itself known is speech. The right side is much more subtle. It works on hunches and intuition.

Linda: This is very interesting, but how does it play into eating?

Bobbe: Very dramatically. I found that one way in which I can change my behavior, because sometimes I cannot change it with clear intent, is by using the right side of my brain to assist me. Just using logic and saying that I am going to lose ten pounds is not enough. It doesn't work. What does seem to work is to take ten minutes a day, sit down, relax, and visualize the weight I want to be. When you see it clearly in front of your eyes you are making an imprint on the right side of your brain. After you see it, you repeat certain affirmations which engage both the left and the right side together. A good one I use is, "I will allow myself to obtain, maintain, and sustain my ideal weight of X pounds by such-and-such a date." You know that trick Weight Watchers members use where you get a picture of a body you like, you paste your face on it, and stare at it several times a day? Well, it works. It gives a message to the right brain.

Linda: I know personally that this method works. I have pictures pasted all around my house. It helps to keep me focused on my goal.

Bobbe: That's right. So many of our actions are habituated responses. We don't even think about what we eat when we eat. It's unconscious. That is why writing it down and making it part of the conscious mind is so important. You must engage both sides of the brain, the conscious left and the unconscious right. You need to change those subtle patterns that have crept in which you are unaware of. It's like that TV commercial, "I can't believe I ate the whole thing." There's another one, too, "I bet you can't eat just one." I know I don't know a piece of See's candy. I know a pound, a box, a bag, but not one piece. I'm better off not to have any. I am better controlled now and if I've run my five miles and have really burned up a lot of calories, I go ahead and have a handful of M & M's and enjoy every bite. But this took years to control. I think it's very important that women understand that weight management is for life. It's not difficult. It takes time and dedication but it is not hard. I say, "Fake it till you make it." Pretend as if you like what you're doing and eventually you will. We're all creatures of habit. Let's just create new habits, make new grooves in our brain.

Linda: I know you strongly believe in using visualization techniques to help people lose weight. Will you explain, step by step, how to do it?

Bobbe: In the morning, first thing if you can, find a quiet place. Sit in a straight-backed chair and get comfortable. I think it's good to begin with a deep breathing technique. My favorite is to inhale eight counts, hold four, and exhale eight, hold four. Do about four or five rounds. Then, say to yourself, "I am relaxed. I am in control." And after about three to four minutes, begin to visualize your body the way you want to be, wearing the clothes you want to, and so on. Be aware that during this time your left brain is going to interfere. It will say to you, "Don't forget to go to the store. We're out of milk. My butt's getting tired. I wonder how long it's been." The best way to handle this is to say, "Thank you. I hear what you're saying. I understand and now I'm going back to my visualizations." Always thank your left brain because you don't want to turn it off completely. If you smell smoke, you want to know it. It is our survival mechanism, so respect it. As you practice this daily, it will take you less time to get relaxed and you will actually have more time for your visualizations. After you get the hang of it, you can add auditory suggestions to your mental pictures. Some I suggest are: "I will allow myself; I know I can; I will; I commit to this as part of my life." When people do this, it makes an incredible impact on their lives—if they do it.

Linda: Is this a type of hypnotism?

Bobbe: In a way. I prefer to call it autosuggestion. This is a naturally occurring state that we undergo several times a day. For example, how many times have we been driving for a distance only to find we have missed our turn? Or read a page in a book and not remembered a word? Our minds were someplace else. We constantly shift into automatic when doing anything that bores the left brain or does not offer a challenge.

The wonderful reality of all this is that whenever we allow the conscious mind, the left brain, the reasonable side of us, to subside long enough for the right brain, the visual, creative side, the unconscious mind, to have the limelight, then we truly tap into the "how to" in reprogramming ourselves. Even if logically you don't think this exercise will make a difference, it doesn't matter. In reality, just practicing it changes behavior.

PART III

Choosing for Better Health

Chapter 12

―――――――――― ❧ ――――――――――

Nourishing the Body

> There is a definite tendency in our culture
> towards self-destructive behavior and living
> the "good life" despite dire consequences.
> —Kenneth R. Pelletier, *Holistic Medicine*

GOOD FOOD MEANS GOOD HEALTH

In our search for health, beauty, and long life, we look in obscure places, or put our faith in quacks and snake-oil doctors, hoping to find a miracle cure for our real and imaginary ills. Yet, the surest and safest solution is the most obvious and the closest at hand: feeding and nourishing the body.

What we eat and drink every day plays a dynamic role in the way we look, act, and feel. Whether we feel and appear weary or energized, anxious or elated, sickly or fit, is largely determined by our diet. Our future health, how quickly we age, and whether we will succumb to often-fatal degenerative diseases have been proven to be related directly to our dietary life-style.

The ancients stressed the importance of good food in health. Some 2,500 years ago, physician-teacher Hippocrates admonished his medical students, "Thy food shall be thy remedy." Today's variation on that axiom is "You are what you eat." Whatever the phrase, the point is that how you feed your body relates directly to your health.

Most of us don't think of nutrition as a separate, complete field of knowledge, but it is. It is a biochemical science based on the incontrovertible laws of nature. When these laws are broken, illness results. A great physician, Henry Beiler, based his entire practice on the belief that improper foods cause disease and proper foods cure disease. In his famous book, *Food Is Your Best Medicine*, he writes, "Health is not something bestowed on you by beneficial Nature at birth; it is achieved and maintained only by active participation in well-defined rules of healthful living—rules which you may be disregarding every day."(1) Food is not the only factor involved in healthy living, but it is a significant one.

DIET VERSUS DISEASE

It would appear that the American people are not conforming to the rules designed by nature. Despite the abundance of food in the United States, government studies, nutritional surveys, and medical evaluations reveal shocking statistics:

* Many Americans are deficient in one or more vitamins and/or minerals.
* Iron deficiency is pervasive in three groups: preschoolers, adolescents, and women over 18.(2)
* Of women aged 18–30 years, 66 percent fail to meet the RDA for calcium; after age 35, the proportion increases to 75 percent.(3)
* Life-style (meaning eating and exercise habits) may ultimately account for more than half of all deaths annually in the United States.(4)
* Current dietary trends may lead to malnutrition through undernourishment.(5)

The good news is that these statistics can be reversed by a change in life-style patterns. Many of the killer diseases that we read and hear about daily (heart disease, arthritis, cancer, and diabetes) have been linked in one way or another to diet and daily habits. Interestingly, while these were once labeled "diseases of civilization," because of their high incidence in industrialized societies as contrasted with underdeveloped areas of the world, these same diseases now are referred to as "diseases of choice."

It is well established that disease breeds far in advance of symptomatology. Most of us become concerned about disease only when we are in pain, but disease generally starts unobtrusively, long before we are remotely aware of it. Subtle biochemical changes occur months, even years, before symptoms are noticed. With little notice, cells, tissues, and eventually organs deteriorate. The body initially handles the strain, but when the problem spreads beyond its ability to cope, disease ensues.

In the early stages, the individual feels nothing out of the ordinary, nor do medical tests reveal any malfunction. As the disease progresses, there may be fatigue, headaches, indigestion, or insomnia. At this point, the deficiency may still be difficult to diagnose, because the clues remain nebulous. Only when serious damage has already occurred can a diagnosis be made. Consider, for example, the woman who finds a lump when examining her breasts. We are relieved that she detected it early, but the fact is that it may already have been five years in the making. She has gone past the point of prevention and now requires diagnosis and treatment. This is what nutritionists seek to avoid.

We need to change our frame of reference—we need to concentrate on preventing disease and illness rather than just treating it. For so many life-threatening diseases—osteoporosis, heart disease, and cancer, to name a few—the best and possibly the only real cure is prevention. That voice crying in the wilderness, out there beyond the "civilized" kingdom of the American Medical Association, is not a quack or an eccentric, but a responsible health professional, the holistic practitioner, saying, "Do something about it *before* it does something about you—before it kills you."

Whether or not you contract a disease depends on more than what you do or do not eat. Your genetic makeup may predispose you to certain illnesses. If your mother, sister, or aunt had diabetes, your risk is heightened. Many findings, however, indicate that inherited characteristics exert less influence on our health than the way we live. Not only are there similar genetic patterns within families, there are also similar dietary habits that may contribute more to the "familial weakness" than genetics. Does your family breakfast on doughnuts and coffee, lunch on hamburgers, fries, and cola, and dine on steak followed by dessert?

Breast cancer, the most common cause of cancer deaths among American women as well as women of other affluent Western countries, is one example of nurture taking precedence over nature. Several studies, including some conducted at the Tufts University School of Medicine and the New England Medical Center in Boston, support the theory that a major determinant for breast cancer in American women appears to be the typical American diet.(6) Epidemiological studies as well as other cancer research over the past 20 years seem to confirm that women from Western countries have higher rates of breast cancer than women of most other nations because their diet is low in fiber and high in fat and sugar.

Poor daily habits make you more susceptible to a variety of illnesses. We are all well informed now about the relationships between smoking cigarettes and lung cancer, sugar and diabetes, stress and hypertension, cholesterol and heart disease, fiber and digestive disturbances. Whatever we do on a regular basis—whether it is smoking, drinking coffee, cola, or alcohol, eating inordinate amounts of sugar, or working under stress—can promote and provoke very definite and predictable disease states in susceptible individuals.

Diet (and I use the term loosely, to encompass everything that enters the digestive tract, including drinks, drugs, and smoke) may not be the only factor for a healthy body, but it is an extremely vital one. All that you put into your mouth eventually reaches your body's cells, creating the environment in which they grow, replenish, and, either thrive or struggle to survive.

WHAT DO HEALTHY PEOPLE EAT?

As part of a search to determine what we should do to become healthy, I have looked into societies and groups of people who have achieved this optimum state. In researching the ultimate diet, I found that the most robust people, living the longest number of years, eat foods as varied as the climates from which they come. Laplanders, who live in a bitterly cold climate, eat primarily reindeer meat and suffer none of the degenerative diseases afflicting more prosperous countries. The beautiful Polynesians in the South Pacific thrive on *poi*, made from the root of the taro plant, raw or cooked fish, and an abundance of fresh tropical plants. The Hunzas of the Himalayas in Asia eat mainly whole grains, fresh fruits and vegetables, fresh milk and cheese, and, on occasion, meat, and they are known as the "healthiest people on Earth." In the United States, Mormons show exceedingly low rates of cancer and heart disease. They often grow their own food, eat more cereal, fruit, and vegetables than meat, and refrain from smoking or drinking coffee, tea, or alcohol.

Even though the selections are diverse, there are definite common denominators among the foods eaten by hearty people the world over, and these can help us in determining what we should eat. Dr. Weston Price, D.D.S., author of *Nutrition and Physical Degeneration*, found that population groups who existed on a natural, unadulterated diet displayed superb health and freedom from the "diseases of choice" mentioned earlier. When these more "primitive" people adopted modern eating habits, they contracted the same degenerative diseases of "civilized" countries within a relatively short period of time (ten years on the average).(7)

This is not to suggest that diet, important as it is, is the only factor involved in the long and healthy lives of people in these societies. Other factors should not be neglected as part of the total picture, for example, genetic endowment, physical activity, and stress level.

The eating habits of healthy peoples, whether they come from the jungles of Africa, the mountains of Tibet, the beaches of the South Pacific, or midtown Manhattan, follow two general rules: Their food is of high nutritional value (what nutritionists call "nutrient dense") and their food is unadulterated (not highly processed). The first component of a nutritious diet is nutrient density. Foods that healthy people consume are loaded with vitamins and minerals in their most natural state. They eat foods that are fresh (locally grown and vine-ripened when possible), and raw or lightly cooked. Processed sugars and grains, packaged foods, and commercial additives are generally unknown to them.

The bottom line? Eat whole foods (foods that are as near to the way God created them as possible) and reduce your intake of substitutes that originate in a test tube. This important rule becomes increasingly crucial to our health as we age. With the passing years, cells rebuild more slowly and deteriorate more rapidly. Some nutrients that are not as efficiently absorbed may be required in greater amounts, even though their calories are not. Obviously, we cannot afford to waste our caloric intake on foods that are not going to feed the body properly.

The foods we consume *most of the time* must be high in nutrient density. We all have favorite recipes, snacks, and celebration delights, and I know that there is no way you are going to deny yourself grandma's famous apple pie forever. As long as these foods are not a daily indulgence, a healthy body will be able to handle them.

For most of us in the United States, over the past 40 years our priorities have become reversed. The balance of what we eat swings more and more toward nonessential rather than essential foods. It is estimated that up to 80 percent of what the majority of Americans eat has no nutritive value whatsoever. No wonder, then, that the American way of life has been called a "high-risk factor" in several diseases. The Senate Select Committee on Nutrition reports that the Standard American Diet (SAD) is high in fat, sugar, and calories, and low in fiber and nutrients. To continue this way of eating, when it is *known* to promote high blood pressure, heart disease, digestive disturbances, skin problems, obesity, blood sugar imbalances, and accelerated aging is indeed SAD. Several leading nutritionists and the Senate Committee have proposed a more nutritious diet plan (see Figure 8). If you are at risk for any of the health problems listed above, it is important that you analyze exactly what you are eating. Consider your daily menus: Are the foods you normally eat high in nutrient density? High in fiber? Low in fat? Low in additives (sugar, salt, unnecessary chemicals)? There is less chance for error if, when you choose your foods, you keep these "basic four" nutrition groups in mind (see Figure 9).

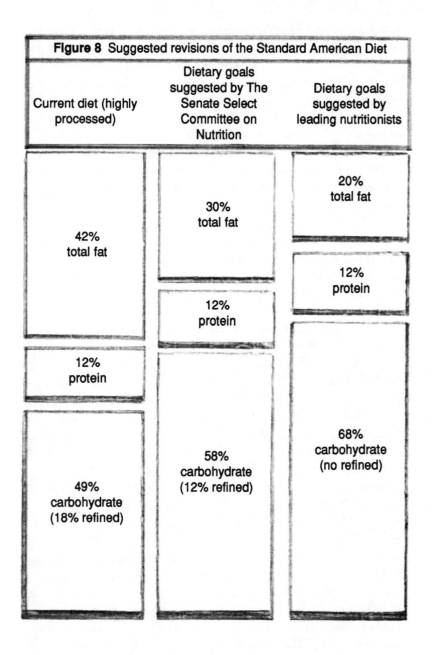

Figure 8 Suggested revisions of the Standard American Diet

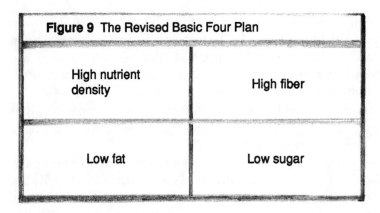

Figure 9 The Revised Basic Four Plan

High nutrient density	High fiber
Low fat	Low sugar

WHEN TO SUPPLEMENT

The question I hear most often when I address groups about nutrition is, "Do I need to supplement my diet with additional vitamins and minerals when I normally eat a balanced diet?" My standard answer is, "It all depends upon your genetic makeup, your diet, your life-style, and your individual symptoms." Too often, we lump people into one group, call them "average," and proceed to make generalized recommendations on a variety of topics. In the area of health this may not be wise, because we are all different.

If we think in terms of "average" or "normal," we might mistakenly believe that we are receiving adequate nourishment. A better description of the "average" person—if we wish to think of ourselves that way—is found in the authoritative *Heinz Handbook of Nutrition*: "The typical individual is more likely to be one who has average needs with respect to many essential nutrients, but who also exhibits some nutritional requirements for a few essential nutrients which are far from average."

Human beings are not genetically uniform. They vary in body frame, weight, dietary preferences, the amount of exercise they take, their digestion and absorption of nutrients, and their ways of dealing with stress. The nutritional requirements of healthy people can vary from "normal" by a factor of as much as 30; those of sick people may vary by factors as high as 1,000.(8)

This diversity, both biochemical and nutritional, is even greater among women. Consider that some women have no children, some have one child, others have fourteen. There are women who nurse their babies for several months, women who are on the pill, women who have had tubal ligations, women who have had partial or radical hysterectomies. Each situation may and usually does require greater than "average" amounts of specific nutrients. When factors vary so dramatically, it is especially difficult if not impossible to formulate "standard" or "average" nutritional requirements.

Many people are born with or develop a need for larger quantities of some nutrients. Andrew Weil, author of *Health and Healing*, explains that our bodies have one or more weak points. Some people are prone to sore throats, others may have sensitive stomachs. Your diet may exacerbate this condition. Nowhere is this clearer than in the case of calcium and its relationship to osteoporosis. Many women inherit a predisposition to osteoporosis; others are at risk because of a lack of calcium in their diet or because of life-style habits that prevent calcium absorption. Whatever the case, increased calcium intake can significantly reduce bone loss in the midlife years.

What confuses many people about nutritional recommendations is the fact that there are always stories of individuals who beat the statistics. Why doesn't everyone who smokes get lung cancer when the research so clearly shows a direct correlation between the two? Obviously, some fortunate individuals have strong constitutions, or above-average respiratory systems.

The question you need to ask yourself is not "Am I average?" but "Do I have a weakness?" If so, you should choose your diet to compensate for that weakness.

Women in general tend to be low in both iron and calcium. Other conditions may indicate greater requirements for certain nutrients. You should consider supplements if you are

* on a diet of fewer than 1,000 calories per day;
* on a fad diet that restricts a major food group;
* pregnant, which usually indicates a need for additional iron and folic acid;
* taking medications (diuretics and some hypertensive drugs deplete potassium; cholestyramine causes poor

absorption of fat, vitamins A, B-12, D, and the minerals iron and potassium; mineral oil and other laxatives cause a loss of vitamins A and D and the mineral calcium; and broad-spectrum antibiotics may decrease vitamin K and some of the B-complex vitamins);

* diagnosed as having a disease in which diet is a recognized factor: hypertension, heart disease, cancer, kidney disease, ulcers, alcoholism; or

* a burn patient, or suffering from a prolonged illness.

If you are a reasonably healthy individual with reasonably healthy parents, a positive outlook on life, and a regular exercise program, and if you maintain your ideal weight, eat a variety of nutrient-rich foods, and avoid excesses of fat, sugar, salt, and alcohol, then you probably do not need additional nutrient reserves. On the other hand, if you do have a physiological weakness or predisposition to a problem and ignore it, you are probably harming your body. Although it is sometimes true that "what you don't know can't hurt you," in this instance, it just may.

Chapter 13

———————— ❧ ————————

Accentuate the Positive

Life is a banquet, but most poor suckers are starving to death.

— Auntie Mame

Nutritionists never agree on what constitutes an optimum diet for two reasons: (i) much of nutrition is not completely understood, and (ii) the optimum is different for every individual. But certain general principles are understood, agreed upon, and can be applied to creating an individual program. An optimum diet would allow the development of an individual to his or her fullest potential, promote the best mental and physical performance, afford the greatest resistance to infection and disease, and not accelerate the aging process. These goals are widely accepted, so, to start a program, let's fill in the dietary basics that also enjoy general acceptance.

PROTEIN

Getting enough protein is not a problem for most American women, unless they are crash dieting on grapefruit and lettuce leaves or consistantly grabbing fast foods in place of meals.

Nutritionists generally recommend 0.8 gram of protein for every two pounds of your ideal body weight. Thus, if you weigh 120 pounds, 48 grams of protein is the amount you require to build, repair, and maintain your cells. The following list translates this into practical measurements.

Are You Getting Adequate Protein?

Food (portion)	Protein Content
beef (3 oz.)	23 g
lamb (3 oz.)	22 g
chicken (3 oz.)	28 g
fish (3 oz.)	21 g
tuna (3 oz.)	24 g
eggs (2)	14 g
milk (1 cup)	9 g
cottage cheese (1/2 cup)	14 g
cheddar cheese (3 oz.)	21 g
beans—1/2 cup	7 g
beans with rice (1 cup)	17 g
vegetarian lasagne (1 cup)	14 g
rice pudding (1 cup)	17 g
wheat cereal and milk (1 cup)	28 g
whole wheat bread (1 slice)	3 g
cornbread (4" x 3")	4 g

We all know that protein is basic to life. Next to water, it is the most plentiful substance in the body, constituting 18–20 percent of body weight. Protein is the structural material that supports the cells, skin, hair, muscles, internal organs, and blood vessels. It builds cells during times of growth and repairs them in emergency situations.

Many substances basic to life functions are made out of protein. Three that stand out are enzymes, antibodies (which help fight foreign bacteria and infection), and hormones (chemical messengers involved in nearly every internal reaction).

Here in the United States we have a rather empirical approach to diet. Because we are a relatively young country, with a wide mix of national origins, we do not have a strong "tradition-al" diet. So we tend to experiment a great deal, trying to sort out the good from the not so good. This also means that when some-thing proves to be good for our health, we have a strong tendency to go overboard. This certainly has happened with protein. For many years, a high-protein diet was the rage. Scores of individuals suffered dangerous side effects; some even sustained irreversible damage to their organs. Important as protein is to the maintenance of the body, an excess is not beneficial and may even cause serious problems. For example:

* Some meats, especially red meats (beef, pork, lamb) are particularly high in fat. High-fat diets are known to promote obesity, hypertension, atherosclerosis, and cancer.

* Red meats aggravate PMS and menstrual cramps.

* Red meats are high in phosphates, which increase the loss of calcium from the bones, creating a greater risk of osteoporosis.

* Large amounts of protein put a strain on the kidneys as they form and excrete organic compounds con-taining nitrogen waste.

* Too much protein may deplete vitamins B-6 and B-3 (pyridoxine and niacin, respectively), calcium, and magnesium.

* Processed and smoked meats such as bacon, ham, salami, and luncheon meats contain nitrates and nitrites, which can lead to the formation of cancer-causing nitrosamines in the body.

Most cuts of meat contain nearly as much fat as protein and possibly even more. A slice of lean ham or a choice grade of slight-ly marbled sirloin is approximately 25 percent protein and 75 per-cent fat. Poultry is generally lower in fat and calories, providing, of course, that you remove the skin and don't fry it.

The meat and poultry raised in developed countries such as the United States contain synthetic hormones, antibiotics, pes-ticide residues, and several other undesirable chemical additives.

Fortunately, in some areas of the country now poultry products are available that have been raised untreated.

Fish is lower in fat than meat and poultry, yet still high in protein. Unless you fry the fish, bread it, or smother it in sauce, the fat content remains very low. Of course, it is best to buy fresh fish, but even canned tuna (packed in water), shrimp, and crab are good sources of protein.

Meat, fish, eggs, and all dairy products provide what nutritionists call "complete" proteins. Each contains all eight essential amino acids or building blocks of protein.

Protein is found in varying amounts in other foods: vegetables, grains, beans, peas, seeds, and nuts. Because they lack or are low in one or more essential amino acids, they are considered incomplete; it is necessary to combine them with complementary foods to produce the complete amino acid configuration.

Though research on proteins and amino acids is quite recent, cultures all over the world have been combining proteins naturally, probably since the dawn of history. Latin Americans thrive on rice and beans. Corn tortillas and beans are a staple among Mexicans. Traditional dishes in the southeastern United States include corn bread and crowder peas, red beans, and rice. In Chinese cuisine, tofu is added to vegetables and rice to make a complete meal.

Three basic food combinations, as explained by Frances Moore Lappe in *Diet for a Small Planet*, form complete proteins and serve as excellent meat substitutes.(1)

* grains (cereal, pasta, rice, or corn) and legumes (beans, peas, or lentils)
  Examples: beans and rice, wheat bread with baked beans, peanut butter sandwich on whole wheat bread, pea soup and toast, legume soup with bread, tortillas, or chappatis

* grains and milk products
  Examples: rice pudding, macaroni and cheese, pasta with cheese, cereal with milk, cheese sandwich, rice and cottage cheese

  * seeds (sesame or sunflower) and legumes (beans,
    peas, or lentils)
    Examples: sesame seeds in bean soups and casseroles,
    sunflower seeds and peanuts, green salad with gar-
    banzo beans, peas, and sunflower seeds, hummus,
    tabouli.

Dairy products are not only useful as accompaniments to
grains, they are excellent by themselves. Milk has been called "the
perfect food" because its amino acid balance matches that of meat,
fish, and poultry. As with other protein sources, those lowest in fat
are preferred: nonfat milk, low-fat cottage cheese, low-fat yogurt,
buttermilk, kefir, and cheeses such as mozzarella, bakers' cheese,
gammelost, krutt, pot, sapsago, and farmers cheese. The most
popular cheeses—Swiss, cheddar, Muenster, Longhorn—are high-
est in fat. Since one ounce of these cheeses contains between 9 and
11 grams of fat, they should be used sparingly.

Milk isn't for everyone, however. Some people are allergic to
milk products, and others may lack the enzyme needed to digest
the lactose or milk sugar (lactose intolerance). If drinking milk or
eating processed cheese causes diarrhea, indigestion, or flatulence,
try fermented milk alternatives (yogurt, kefir, buttermilk, or acidophilus milk). If the digestive difficulties continue, omit dairy
products completely from your diet. There are enough proteins
available from other sources; if you are concerned about your calcium intake, you can always take a supplement.

Seeds and nuts are best eaten fresh and raw, and are a rich
source of protein and fiber. They can be eaten alone as a snack or
combined in a meal for added nutrients, flavor, and texture.
Power-still packed as they are, it is best not to go overboard unless
you can afford the calories. A half-cup of peanuts or walnuts contains 36 grams of fat.

An increasingly popular protein source is tofu, the tradition-
al East Asian food product made from soybeans. It is close in nutritional quality to meat protein and is an excellent complement to
grains. Tofu has little or no taste, and takes on the flavor of the ac-
companying foods. I prefer it prepared Japanese style—mixed with
stir-fried vegetables over rice. Since tofu is easy to digest and low

in fats, cholesterol, and calories, it is recommended for those who cannot eat fat-rich meat and are sensitive to dairy foods.

CARBOHYDRATES

Carbohydrates are supposedly synonymous with weight gain, and are therefore shunned like the plague by many women. The fact is, once your daily quota of calories has been filled, by any food group, whether carbohydrates, fats, or proteins, *any* excess is stored as fat. Thus, all foods are fattening if eaten in excess.

Actually, the body "runs" on carbohydrates: They are the only true clean-burning fuel in the diet. Both protein and fat release toxic by-products as the body metabolizes them. Carbohydrates do not; in fact they temper the toxins. That is why a diet high in protein and fat and low in carbohydrates can overburden the organs and decrease your energy. Athletes and exercise freaks, take note: Carbohydrates, especially complex carbohydrates, are the best available source of energy.

Since complex carbohydrates (found in whole grains, beans, rice, fruits, and vegetables) are rich in nutrients, are a great source of fiber, are low in fat, and can double as protein, they can potentially serve our total dietary needs. Vegetarians have long proven that fact. The Senate Select Committee on Nutrition recommends that they consitute the bulk of our diet. A well-planned carbohydrate meal fulfills all of the "revised basic four" diet requirements (see Figure 9 in Chapter 12).

THE ROLE OF FIBER

The principal carbohydrates present in foods are sugar, starches, and fiber. Sugars and starches basically provide the body with energy. Dietary fiber, on the other hand, has several different roles.

There are two kinds of fiber: insoluble and soluble. Water-insoluble fiber, found in wheat bran and some fruits and vegetables, attracts water to the digestive tract, thereby softening the stool and helping to prevent constipation. It also exercises the muscles of the digestive system, which in turn, keeps the intestines toned and more resistant to diverticulosis.

Soluble fiber, found in high concentration in oat bran, beans, and many fruits and vegetables, is made up of microscopic particles that travel through the blood stream picking up fat. Soluble fiber has proven to be effective in lowering both cholesterol and triglyceride levels in the blood, thereby reducing the risk of heart disease.

Many people can benefit from adding fiber to the diet. It has been found that diabetics have been able to reduce their insulin requirements by adding more fiber to their diets because it appears to modulate levels of blood sugar after eating. Dieters too can be helped by eating more fibrous foods. Foods such as fruits, vegetables, beans, and whole grains take longer to chew and add bulk to a meal, both of which help a dieter to feel full.

Obviously, fibrous foods have numerous health benefits. One I haven't mentioned is their contribution of vitamins and minerals to the body. For example, whole-grain flours are rich in B vitamins and protein; fruits give us vitamin C and many minerals; vegetables are high in vitamin A and also minerals.

There are many things you could do to increase the amount of fiber in your diet. Below are just a few suggestions.

* Switch to a high-fiber bread, such as sprouted wheat, wheat berry, or 100% whole grain.

* Have a high-fiber cold cereal for breakfast three to four times a week such as Bran Flakes, Bran Chex, Raisin Bran, or Cracklin' Oat Bran.

* Make a high-fiber soup once a week: bean soup, lentil soup, corn chowder, cabbage soup, or vegetable soup with beans.

* Use beans in your green salads: chick-peas (garbanzo beans), green beans, kidney beans, or peas.

* Make vegetable dishes that contain beans, such as three-bean salad, succotash, rice with peas, or broccoli with kidney beans.

* Eat high-fiber vegetables every day, including corn, broccoli, brussels sprouts, spinach, peas, green beans, potatoes.

* Serve fruit as often as possible, including blueberries, strawberries, pears, raisins, bananas, and apples.
* Use dark-green salad greens, such as spinach, romaine, and endive, instead of pale iceberg lettuce.
* Try bean dips served with chili or raw vegetables, or whole-wheat pita bread.
* Purchase unprocessed wheat bran and All-Bran for use in regular recipes for pies, cakes, and cookies.
* Add unprocessed wheat and oat bran to meat loaf, casseroles, and vegetable dishes as an extender or make crumb toppings for baked fruit desserts.
* Eat corn, bran, or oat muffins instead of cakes, doughnuts, and cookies.
* Add raisins to muffins, cereal, rice pudding, and cookies.
* Use part whole-wheat, soy, or oat flour in your standard recipes.
* Snack on whole-grain crackers and dried fruits.
* Use nuts and seeds in recipes.

FAT

About 40 percent of the calorie intake in the average American diet comes from fats and oils. This is equivalent to about three ounces of fat or three-quarters of a stick of butter per person per day. Surprised? Do you conscientiously trim the fat off your meat and resist eating bread and butter? Are you convinced someone else—not you—is making up this "average"? The problem is that most of us are unaware of how many fats are camouflaged in our foods. How often do we eat the following: fast foods, TV dinners, take- out delicatessen sandwiches, hot dogs, luncheon meats, peanut butter, bread, crackers, nuts, potato chips, corn chips, avocados, cheese, quiche, salad dressing, pizza, rice pudding, potato salad, paté, pastries, mousse, croissants, dips, doughnuts, ice cream, cheesecake, cream soups, sauces, carrot cake, pie, cookies, and chocolate? These are all high in fat.

A high-fat diet contributes to obesity. Fat has over twice the calories of both protein and carbohydrates: nine calories per gram compared to four calories per gram for the other two (alcoholic beverages contain seven calories per gram). A high-fat diet contributes to a raft of common health problems: high blood pressure, heart disease, diabetes, and breast cancer. Reducing overall fat consumption to 30 percent or, better yet, 20 percent of your diet should be your long-term goal.

There are three kinds of fats in food: saturated, polyunsaturated, and monounsaturated. Saturated fats are generally solid at room temperature and come primarily from animal products such as red meat, poultry (especially the skin), whole milk, cheese, butter, and cream. Since saturated fats have been found to raise blood cholesterol levels, many people have become more conscious of reducing these foods in their diets. What is not as well known is that some widely used vegetable oils are also saturated, and thus carry with them the same potential risks. Both palm kernel and coconut oil are highly saturated—in fact, even more saturated than beef fat. These oils are commonly used by manufacturers in making every variety of snacks imaginable, from crackers and chips to cookies, cakes, whipped dessert toppings, and granola bars.

Polyunsaturated fats are generally liquid at room temperature and are derived from vegetable sources such as corn, safflower, and soybean. Except for coconut and palm oils, these oils are not saturated and have been shown to lower blood cholesterol levels.

Monosaturated fats are derived from olives, peanuts, and avocados. Recent evidence indicates that they too lower total blood cholesterol.

Reducing saturated fats in the diet should be a concern to all of us in terms of lowering risk factors for many diseases. This does not mean that you can eat as many polyunsaturated fats as you like. All fats have more than twice the calories per gram than either proteins or carbohydrates. In other words, fats make you fat. Dietary fats are converted more efficiently into body fats than either protein or carbohydrates, and the body expends fewer calories to metabolize them than it does for the other two. If you are concerned about your weight, consume fewer total fats.

Tips for Reducing Fat Content in Your Diet

* Cut down on red meats; use them as a side dish rather than as a main course.
* Buy leaner cuts of meat, such as round steak, flank steak, and lean ground sirloin.
* Trim all visible fat from meat before cooking.
* Replace red meats with turkey and chicken—particularly the white meat.
* Skin poultry before cooking.
* Choose fish more often—especially scrod, flounder, cod, haddock, shrimp, lobster, red snapper, and tuna (packed in water).
* Bake, broil, or stir fry rather than deep fry.
* Experiment with nonmeat dinners once or twice a week.
* Decrease use of oil and butter in cooking and baking.
* Minimize cheese, sauces, and dips, and use low-fat substitutes when you can (nonfat milk, plain yogurt, cottage cheese).
* Limit use of seeds, nuts, and avocados if weight is a problem.
* Eliminate processed and packaged foods completely.
* Watch intake of desserts—especially pies, doughnuts, chocolate, ice cream, and other creamy, gooey concoctions.

WATER

An often overlooked ingredient in the good health and energy equation is water. Next to oxygen, it is the most important nutrient we can give our bodies. A healthy adult can survive for weeks without food, but only days without water. A loss of even 10 percent of total body fluid is serious.

Water is essential to all living organisms. It is the major constituent of body fluid, making up about half of the body weight in an average adult female and about 60 percent in the adult male.

This percentage varies inversely with the fat content of the body; thus, when less fat is present (as is the case with men), water is a greater percentage of the body weight.

Water is absolutely essential to blood building and internal cleansing, to the proper functioning of the kidneys and sweat glands, and to our entire digestive process. It facilitates the transportation of nutrients and hormones to the cells and flushes toxic wastes out of the body. People who drink a lot of water seldom have elimination problems.

In addition to transporting molecules of oxygen and hydrogen to the cells, water is also, in itself, a source of minerals that are particularly important to the blood, bones, and heart. Several studies in both the United States and the United Kingdom have found that rates of death from heart disease are generally lower in regions where people drink mineralized "hard" water. Soft water may be great for laundry, but its lack of calcium and magnesium in addition to its high sodium content make it a poor choice for drinking.

Many people mistakenly feel they are consuming their quota of liquid because they continually drink coffee, tea, soda pop, and diet drinks. Even though these beverages are water based, the pure water has been corrupted with syrup, caffeine, and chemical additives. Instead of hydrating the system, these draw the water out; instead of cleansing, they pollute and burden the dried-out organs; instead of quenching, they cause thirst.

As we age, we naturally lose about 10–15 percent of our body fluid. If we compound this loss by continually dehydrating our bodies with coffee, sugar, and alcohol, we are likely to wrinkle and age prematurely. For moist mucous membranes on the inside and plump-looking wrinkle-free skin on the outside, we must drink a lot of fresh water.

Certain foods contain a great deal of water and are refreshing, cleansing, and energizing. More than 90 percent of juicy fruits and vegetables such as tomatoes, lettuce, cauliflower, eggplant, watermelon, and strawberries are water. Whole milk is 87 percent water; avocados, bananas, and sweet potatoes contain 75 percent water; and, strangely enough, many kinds of low-fat fish are a fair source of water.

However, we can't depend on foods to fill our need for fluid. An average person, of average build, should drink 6–8 8-ounce glasses of pure spring or bottled water each day—more if it's hot, if he or she is exercising, if he or she is having hot flushes, and (believe it or not) if he or she is bloated or retaining water.

The foods we eat and the fluids we drink all work together in creating good health. High-quality proteins and fibrous carbohydrates low in saturated fat provide the raw materials necessary for a healthy body.

Chapter 14

———————— ❧ ————————

Eliminate the Negative

> Every day you do one of two things: build
> health or produce disease in yourself.
> — Adelle Davis

NONFOODS

As I said in Chapter 13 in the discussion about grains, to choose healthful foods, look for those that are as close to their original, whole state as possible. This means avoiding foods whose natural integrity has been violated. Foods created in a laboratory cannot match the nutritional quality of a natural product. Even if they have been carefully designed to incorporate several vitamins and minerals, they do not contain the mysterious micronutrients— enzymes and trace minerals—that have yet to be discovered and duplicated. For these elusive elements, we need "real" food. This is why most nutritionists prefer foods to pills as the source of nutrients.

Almost all reports and research indicate that the health and longevity of a population are related to the naturalness and wholesomeness of the foods they eat. In cultures where the diet consists totally of fresh, whole, unprocessed, and unrefined foods, people (if they get enough to eat) enjoy good health, long life, and a relative absence of disease. Once their diet changes to include denatured, refined, human-made foods, disease creeps in, and people lose their seemingly mysterious secret of life and good health.

Virtually all supermarket food today contains chemicals that were added either in the growing stage or later, during processing. Long before most foods reach manufacturers, they are treated with fertilizers, herbicides, and pesticides, injected with hormones, tranquilizers, and antibiotics, or exposed to the chemical wastes of industrial society. Later, on the production line, as a food is prepared and packaged, it may be treated with any number of additional chemicals, some of which may be harmful. For example, a group of acknowledged carcinogens (cancer-causing agents)— sodium nitrate and sodium nitrite—are routinely used to preserve luncheon meats, hot dogs, smoked fish, bacon, and ham. There is no question that these additives produce a cancer-causing substance, yet they continue to be used. Each one is present supposedly in quantities small enough to be harmless.

To list all the pollutants and poisons found in processed foods would take a book in itself. There are literally thousands, disguised as stabilizers, imitation flavors, thickeners, softeners, emulsifiers, sweeteners, bleaches, enhancers, conditioners, ripeners, waxes, acidifiers—and the list goes on. Yet many research studies show that when taken together, interacting, they may not be harmless at all, and that we—or the manufacturers—may be playing Russian roulette with our lives and health. It may shock you to know that each of us supposedly consumes about five pounds of these additives per year. The long-term effects of many of them are still unknown, as are the cumulative consequences of a lifetime of ingesting these substances.

The food industry determined long ago that these substances are necessary to maintain shelf life, to preserve the appearance or enhance the appeal of a product. There is little chance it will stop using them in the interest of better nutrition: Large-scale production has always been motivated by profits rather than health. As consumers we have two choices: We can vow never to eat a food that has been "adulterated" (eliminating, of course, just about everything at the grocery store), or we can be prudent in our selection of products, taking the time to read and compare labels. In time, if enough consumers select foods with fewer additives, the food industry will respond and start reducing, perhaps even eliminating, the additives in their products. One more safeguard is to eat a variety of foods, which reduces the risk of getting too much of a particular additive.

SUGAR

Two food additives deserve honorable or, to be more accurate, dishonorable mention because they are so terribly overused in the Western diet. Since both sugar and salt are relatively inexpensive, they are used extensively by the food industry to preserve, flavor, and extend the shelf life of many products. If you think your diet is relatively low in sugar, go into your pantry and inspect the labels. Sugar, disguised in its many different forms as dextrose, sucrose, fructose, maltose, corn syrup, beet sugar, honey, and molasses, probably appears on all your product labels: canned fruits and vegetables, yogurt, salad dressing, pickles, catsup, toothpaste, antacids, and cough medicine. Many items contain more than one form of sugar, so you can be sure you are getting better than your fair share. Believe it or not, most Americans individually consume 140 pounds of sugar per year.

As we approach menopause we require fewer calories, but the same amount of nutrients. We need to minimize foods that not only lack nutritive value but also destroy the nutrients we have consumed. At the top of the list of such foods is sugar. How bad is sugar? So bad that not even a lowly microbe can survive in it.

As sugar is metabolized, it drains the body of many vitamins. Unlike natural carbohydrates—such as apples, oranges, and whole grains—refined white sugar enters the body unaccompanied by the team of nutrients needed to facilitate its digestion and assimilation. These nutrients are leached out of our body's resources, and, over time, tapping into our body's reserves creates multiple deficiencies, especially within the B-complex family. As a result, most women with a sweet tooth are deficient in B vitamins. Initial signs of such deficiency are relatively minor: fatigue, water retention, anxiety, irritability, and depression. Long-term deficiencies, however, may have serious consequences. Studies at McGill

Medical School have determined that there is a direct correlation between B-vitamin deficiency and estrogen-based cancers.(1) In the absence of adequate B vitamins, estrogen builds up and is subsequently stored in the estrogen receptors of the breast and uterus. A vicious cycle results: As the production of estrogen increases, the deficiency becomes more pronounced; the greater the deficiency, the more estrogen is secreted.

Sugar induces considerable alterations in the levels of several hormones as they attempt to maintain a chemical balance within the body. The pancreas, liver, and adrenal glands are all overstimulated by fluctuation in blood-sugar levels. While our bodies can handle blood-sugar highs and lows in our youthful years, the day of reckoning comes when the system loses its resilience.

For menopausal women, symptoms of this change may be related to the inability of the worn-out adrenal glands to take over estrogen production as the ovaries decline. When the glands are strong and healthy, they are much more capable of secreting adequate amounts of estrogen to prevent dramatic hormonal fluctuations, which have been related to menopausal symptoms.

Probably the most critical problem women face, both before and during menopause, is getting and absorbing enough calcium to prevent osteoporosis. Sweet eaters beware! Sugar inhibits calcium absorption. To guard against the most devastating of all menopausal problems—brittle bones—watch your sugar now.

A sweet tooth, like any bad habit or addiction, can be brought under control if one is truly motivated. For some women, conscious awareness is enough to make the change. For others who have become physically addicted to sugar, there may actually be withdrawal symptoms when it is eliminated. Approach the change with care, planning, self-love, and patience. To retrain your taste buds will take time and effort. Go slowly. Don't try to reverse 30 years of indiscriminate eating in two days, or two weeks.

Everyone asks for advice on how to handle sugar cravings. I recommend that you concentrate on the specific micronutrients affected by eating sugar: the B vitamins, magnesium, chromium, zinc, and manganese. Foods rich in these key substances include certain fruits and vegetables, whole grains, and wheat germ. But don't wait until you have given in to the desire for a double hot-fudge sundae to start suddenly eating greens. Prepare your body in advance by keeping it well nourished and well supplied.

Artificial sweeteners are not the best alternative to sugar, although they may be temporarily useful. Saccharine, cyclamates, and aspartame have all been linked to cancer and various side effects. To replace one potential enemy with another is hardly a satisfactory resolution of a conflict. What we ultimately need to do is to retrain the hunger or expectation of our taste buds for sweetness.

You're probably wondering about the value of raw sugar, molasses, carob, and honey—the so-called natural sugars. Bad news: All forms of sugar deplete the nutrient supply and cause a sudden elevation in the blood sugar, that is, in the amounts we normally eat. Unlike table sugar or sucrose, however, these more respected natural sweeteners do have some nutritional value: Carob is rich in B vitamins and minerals; honey contains small amounts of trace minerals and traces of the vitamins B, C, D, and E; molasses is high in iron, calcium, copper, magnesium, phosphorus, pantothenic acid, inositol, and vitamins B and E. If you must use a sweetener for baking or on your cereals, the natural ones are slightly better. Just try to use them sparingly.

Why Women Must Control Their Cravings for Sweets

* Sugars are a nonnutritive nonfood.
* They deplete vitamin and mineral stores, especially vitamins B and C and the minerals magnesium and chromium.
* They create hormone fluctuations and imbalances, aggravating menstrual problems.
* They cause extremes in blood-sugar levels.
* They create stress for the endocrine glands (adrenals, pancreas).
* They trigger hot flashes.
* They inhibit calcium absorption, and thus can contribute to osteoporosis.
* They are addictive.

* They have been linked to obesity, digestive disturbances, tooth decay, diabetes, increased blood
  cholesterol and triglyceride levels, and urinary tract
  infections.

TABLE SALT (SODIUM CHLORIDE)

Sodium chloride has been used for a long time to preserve food.
Unlike simple sugar, however, sodium is an essential nutrient. It is
required for the maintenance of blood volume, the regulation of
fluid balance, the transport of molecules across the cell wall, and
the transmission of impulses along nerve fibers.

Recent government studies indicate, however, that most
Americans consume far more salt than is necessary. Daily, we are
told, we take in, on the average, between 6 and 20 grams of sodium
chloride; we need no more than 1 to 3 grams per day. To satisfy our
real need for salt, we need no more than is found in the foods we
normally eat. Even when no salt is added during cooking or at the
table, the sodium quickly adds up.

Sodium Content of Common Foods

eggs (2 medium)	108 mg
ground beef (1/4 lb.)	76 mg
hamburger (commercial)	950 mg
hot dog	627 mg
haddock (4 oz.)	201 mg
whole-wheat bread (1 slice)	148 mg
corn flakes (1/2 cup)	126 mg
waffle	356 mg
chocolate cake (1 piece)	233 mg
fresh peas	2 mg
canned peas (1/2 cup)	200 mg
potato (1 medium)	6 mg
hash brown potatoes (1/2 cup)	223 mg
milk (1 cup)	128 mg
low-fat cottage cheese (1 cup)	918 mg
cheddar cheese (1 oz.)	176 mg
roquefort cheese (1 oz.)	513 mg

dill pickle	928 mg
commercial salad dressing (1 tbsp.)	219 mg
canned minestrone soup (1 cup)	2,033 mg

Excess, as we all know, is unhealthy. Eating too much salt can raise the blood pressure and, in doing so, increase the risk of heart and kidney disease. Salt stimulates water retention, which is uncomfortable, adds unwanted pounds to the body, and prevents the loss of fat. In the menopausal woman, salt may trigger annoying hot flashes and promote loss of calcium from the bones. The exact amount of calcium loss and bone breakdown caused by high salt intake is not known, but any loss is significant for high-risk women in their middle years.

Sodium can aggravate premenstrual syndrome. Niels Lauersen, M.D., writes that the elimination of salt in the diet alone has helped many PMS sufferers reduce their bloatedness, premenstrual irritability, and headaches.(2) He indicates that it is important for women with PMS to reduce their salt intake greatly during the two weeks preceding their periods, when PMS symptoms can be the worst.

To reduce the amount of salt in your diet, start with the obvious offenders—chips, crackers, ham, bacon, and other smoked or cured meats, processed cheese, and table salt. Then, look for the hidden salt in processed foods. In checking labels, look for anything with the word *sodium* in it, such as monosodium glutamate and sodium nitrate, and watch for the abbreviated chemical symbol *Na*.

Many good books have been written with excellent recipes for a low-salt diet. My favorite is *The American Heart Association Cookbook*. (American Health Association, 1984). Commonly available salt substitutes contain potassium in place of all or part of the sodium. People under medical supervision, particularly for kidney problems, should check with their physicians before using these salt substitutes. Alternatives to salt that contain mixtures of spices and herbs, such as Veg-it, are recommended. You can also substitute for regular table salt with mixed herbs, fresh spices, garlic, lemon juice, and unsalted salad dressing. Be creative, find new tastes you like and explore them. Once you do, you will find it difficult to eat something that is highly salted.

You should also be cautious of what you drink. Soft water, carbonated soda, and some bottled waters contain sodium. Ordinary club soda has 241 mg; Perrier water, 14 mg; and Poland Spring water, 4 mg. Being alert to a significant difference may be more important if you are prone to PMS, water retention, or high blood pressure.

CAFFEINE

Coffee is the most widely used stimulant in the United States. Hidden behind the friendly brown color and delicious aroma of brewing coffee is the stimulant drug, caffeine. This white crystalline alkaloid produces strong physiological effects, some of which we know and desire, and others about which we're uninformed. Caffeine stimulates the central nervous system, warding off fatigue and temporarily giving us the feeling of mental alertness. In some individuals it may create a general sense of well-being, improve reaction time, enhance accuracy, and even enhance endurance. But this is only half the story.

When caffeine is taken in excess—and that limit is a function of individual tolerance—the entire central nervous system is overstimulated. Nervous reactions that result may include shakiness, heart palpitations, chronic anxiety, and dizziness. Menopausal women report that caffeine often triggers hot flashes, sweating, and insomnia.

Caffeine promotes the release of insulin from the pancreas and of adrenalin from the adrenal cortex, raising the blood-sugar level initially to an unnatural high, which eventually drops to an unhealthy low. Contrary to the hopes and dreams of dieters, the insulin response initiated by the stimulant winds up increasing the appetite, enhancing the craving for sweets, and encouraging the storage of fat.

An effective diuretic, coffee forces the excretion of more than normal amounts of water, vitamins, and minerals. The water soluble vitamins B and C are particularly susceptible to forced water loss. Calcium, the mineral so important for healthy bones, can also be lost by drinking too much coffee.

Caffeine has been implicated in the development of fibrocystic breast disease, a benign condition characterized by breast tenderness and lumps. Eliminating caffeine completely has been shown to reduce both the size and painfulness of the lumps in two to six months.(3) As both a coffee lover and a woman with fibrocystic breast pain, I can personally confirm the results of this research. Only one small cup of freshly brewed Colombian coffee will give me pains within the hour.

Caffeine affects the gastrointestinal, cardiovascular, and circulatory systems as well. Shortly after you drink a cup of espresso, your stomach temperature rises, your hydrochloric acid output increases, your heart beats faster, and the blood vessels constrict (narrow) around the brain, yet dilate (widen) around your heart. Your metabolic rate increases, the uric acid in your blood increases, there is reduced blood flow to your extremities, and your eyeball pressure is raised. Anyone suffering from glaucoma should be warned against drinking coffee.

Obviously, the effects of caffeine are systemwide, touching every organ, tissue, and cell in the body. Recently, caffeine has also been linked to the incidence of several cancers; however, more studies are needed to confirm these reports.

A "moderate" dose of caffeine is 2 mg per pound of body weight; thus, if you weigh 130 pounds, it is considered "safe" for you to take in 260 mg of caffeine per day. This isn't very much when you consider that a single cup of coffee contains between 100 and 150 mg of caffeine. Remember, too, that coffee is not the only source of caffeine. It is frequently a major ingredient in over-the-counter diet pills and in prescription drugs for pain, menstrual cramps, allergies, and headaches. Use the following list to determine how much caffeine you may be taking into your body.

Determining Caffeine Levels

Source	Milligrams
coffee (1 cup)	
drip	110–150
percolated	64–124
instant	40–108

tea (1 cup)
    black, brewed 5 min.   20–50
    black, brewed 1 min.   9–33
    instant   12–28
    iced   22–36
soft drinks (12 oz.)
    Coke   46
    Pepsi   41
    Tab   46
    Mountain Dew   54
    Diet Coke   46
chocolate
    milk chocolate (1 oz.)   20–35
    hot chocolate (1 cup)   5–10
drugs
    Excedrin   65
    (Excedrin P.M. has no caffeine)
    Anacin   32
    Midol   32
    Cope   32
    Dexatrim   200
    No Doz   100
    Darvon   32
    Vivarin   100
    aspirin   0

Changing any lifelong pattern can be stressful. Most experts suggest a gradual weaning process, rather than stopping "cold turkey." Because caffeine is a drug, when you stop abruptly you may experience any number of withdrawal symptoms: headaches, drowsiness, nausea, nervousness, depression, indigestion, edema, constipation, cramps, and, strangely, even a runny nose. Give yourself time to make this transition. Taper off by eliminating a few cups a day if you are a heavy coffee drinker. Substitute with decaffeinated coffee some of the time, or try tea or, better yet, herb tea, Postum, juice, mineral water, or plain water with a twist of lemon. Once you have kicked the coffee habit, you will have more natural energy than you did after your four-cup fix of caffeine.

ALCOHOL

Like all the other drugs just mentioned, alcohol provides little or no nutrition, depletes vital nutrients, and places a heavy burden on the hormonal system, the digestive system, and the kidneys. Taken to extremes, alcohol consumption actively damages organs such as the pancreas and the liver, and can disrupt the entire nervous system permanently. It is well established that it increases the risk of diabetes, heart disease, and cancer, and its addictive qualities, for some people, are a nightmare.

Certain women are hypersensitive to alcohol. PMS sufferers have a decreased alcohol tolerance during the days preceding their periods. Even one glass of wine may be enough to cause intoxication.

The potential long-term effects of alcohol consumption are even more frightening. One British study indicates that women who drink regularly have a 1.5–2 times higher rate of breast cancer than those who never drink.(4) Women who both smoke and drink are at an even greater risk, suggesting that there may be an adverse multiple factor in effect when both habits are involved simultaneously.

One explanation for why alcohol may increase the risk of breast cancer is proposed by nutritional biochemist Jeffrey Bland, Ph.D. He believes that it is related to the adverse effect alcohol has on the liver. One function of the liver is to break down estrogen so that it can be excreted safely from the body. "The inability to properly metabolize estrogen can lead to the buildup of certain estrogenic substances within the body that can overly stimulate receptors in the breast, ovary, or uterine wall and initiate a cancer process."(5) As was noted previously, B-vitamin deficiencies can also cause estrogen oversecretion, and alcohol depletes B vitamins.

Over half of the problems associated with excessive long-term alcohol consumption stem from the malnutrition that results from continual use. Alcohol, a derivative of sugar, is metabolized in the body in a similar way. It requires substantial nutrients from other sources or from the body's reserve supply before it can be metabolized, or converted into energy. Thus, it creates deficiencies of the B vitamins, vitamin C, calcium, magnesium, potassium, and zinc.

Any woman at risk for osteoporosis should carefully monitor her alcohol intake. Alcohol impairs calcium absorption and may affect the ability of the liver to activate vitamin D. It is not known how much alcohol it takes to effect significant bone loss; what has been established, though, is the fact that alcoholics are at much greater risk for developing osteoporosis.

Alcohol has also been reported to aggravate the common menopausal symptoms of hot flashes, insomnia, and depression. Since it is high in calories, it easily adds unwanted pounds that build up around the midsection. And as a dehydrating substance, alcohol, in excess, can result in premature wrinkling and loss of skin tone.

Individuals who eat nutritious diets and are in good physical condition can absorb the occasional drink without severe detrimental effects; it can possibly even have positive health benefits. Alcohol in moderation is a social lubricant. It can relieve tension, stimulate the appetite (aperitif), and aid digestion (digestif). As I have said before, it is not what you eat or drink occasionally that will harm you, it's what you put into your body on a regular basis.

Recent reports indicate that one or two ounces of alcohol a day may slightly decrease the risk of heart disease. It appears that this preventive role of alcohol is related to an increase in high-density lipoproteins (HDL)—the fraction of cholesterol that seems to protect against atherosclerosis (hardening of the arteries). I do not advocate drinking alcohol in order to raise your HDLs, however; exercise is every bit as effective and has no side effects.

To a large degree, alcohol tolerance is an individual—or family— matter. If you are hypoglycemic, have a history of breast cancer in your family, are prone to osteoporosis, suffer from hot flashes, depression, insomnia, or PMS, or have a problem with moderate drinking, you probably need to refrain from alcohol completely.

SMOKING

Smoking is the largest single cause of premature death and ill health for women and men in America. A woman who smokes runs twice the risk of dying from a stroke, and eight to twelve times the risk of dying from lung cancer. Because women are now smoking as much as men, they have caught up with men in incidence of lung cancer. Lung cancer is now the number one cancer killer of women, exceeding breast cancer.

The risks of smoking increases with age and the number of years smoked. These risks include osteoporosis, glaucoma, cardiovascular disease, and several kinds of cancer. There is an increased risk of heart disease among women who both take oral contraceptives and smoke, and an increased risk of cancer of the mouth, pharynx, larynx, and esophagus among people who both smoke and drink.

Chapter 15

————————— ❧ —————————

Correcting Deficiencies in Your Diet

Planning is bringing the future into the present so that you can do something about it now.

—Alan Lakein,
How to Get Control of Your Time and Your Life

CHARTING FOR HEALTH

We all know firsthand that what we eat has an immediate effect on how we feel. What we eat and how we live in our younger years may directly determine the quality of our future health. For this reason, we need to analyze our eating and determine if we are adequately prepared.

As we get older, it becomes increasingly important to monitor the quality of food we eat. Physical problems increase because the body cannot produce hormones, enzymes, and antibodies at the same rate and in the same amounts as before. Nutrients are absorbed and utilized less efficiently. To maintain health, we must provide the body with a steady supply of high-grade nutrients, and avoid foods and substances that strain the system.

For some, this may mean embarking on a major program to take charge of their health. The first step is determining where you are and where you want to go. Awareness of the need to change always precedes action, and you should take some time now to understand your own, individualized, particular needs. Before you make any specific dietary alterations, or go out and spend a fortune on supplements, start by analyzing your eating habits, your lifestyle, and your present symptoms.

Before making any changes, check any and every unusual symptom with your family doctor. Even something as seemingly innocuous as fatigue could indicate a serious problem. When you have a clean bill of health, then proceed.

Any new program must begin with the basics, and that is precisely where we are going—back to the most basic substance our body needs: good, wholesome, nutritious food. The first step is to review everything that enters your mouth. The most effective way to do this is by charting—writing down every day for several weeks exactly what you eat and drink.

You could use a very large calendar, such as a desk calendar, or, better yet, buy some poster paper and make your own chart. This will reinforce your serious intent to change your habits. Now, chart your eating patterns for three weeks. Why so long? For several reasons: It is important to record and review different eating situations, such as weekend parties, family get-togethers, lunches out, office meals, and days alone. It is especially important to analyze the week before, during, and after your menstrual period.

See the chart illustrated in Chapter 11; the same kind of charting used in gaining control of your weight is excellent for helping you gain control of your nutrition. Make three columns: a small one for the times of day you eat or snack, a larger one for the food, and another small one for recurring feelings or symptoms. Be specific—for example, write down the *kind* of cereal (oatmeal, cornflakes, or Cocoa Krispies), the *kind* of bread (white, rye, whole-grain wheat), how the food was prepared (fried, broiled, steamed, raw), how *much* you ate. Don't forget condiments: catsup, mustard, mayonnaise, pickles, and so on. In the symptom column, record how you feel; you can use your own system of abbreviations or symbols for your particular problems. Fill in this column as and when your symptoms occur—midmorning, after lunch, and so on.

After a very interesting—and revealing—three weeks, you will be ready for the dietary and life-style test below. It might be easier if you go through your chart and circle specific areas with different colored pens (e.g., sugar foods with red, fatty foods with green, and processed foods with blue). After three weeks have gone by, you will definitely be in tune to your eating habits. Not only will you know the types of foods you eat regularly, but you will also see how often you eat (or don't eat) and how frequently you experience recurring symptoms.

As a cross-check or a quick self-test, you can get a general idea of your dietary habits right now. Go ahead and answer the following questions. Put a check mark next to each item for which your answer is yes.

Dietary and Life-style Analysis

1. Do you frequently (more than 4 times a week) eat

__fast foods

__canned fruits, vegetables, and soups

__fried, breaded, or deep-fried meats or vegetables

__desserts, doughnuts, cupcakes, cookies, pie, ice cream

__packaged or frozen foods, instant products

__white bread, white rice

__hot dogs, bacon, luncheon meats

__chips and crackers

__condiments (catsup, mustard, syrups, jam, mayonnaise)

__candy

2. Do you frequently drink

___coffee—more than 2 cups a day

___soda pop, diet cola, tea, decaffeinated coffee

___alcohol—more than 5 times a week

3. Do you often skip one or more meals?

4. Are you on a diet of less than 1,000 calories per day?

5. Do you smoke?

6. Do you take medication?

7. Are you continually under stress?

8. Are you inactive, having no regular exercise program?

9. Do you have several annoying symptoms (gas, fatigue, headaches, hemorrhoids, insomnia)?

If you checked fewer than five items, your diet is probably healthy. If you checked close to half, you need to make some adjustments in your diet or life-style. If you checked most of the items, you should get a physical and reevaluate your life-style. You definitely need both a drastic change of diet and nutritional reinforcement.

ARE YOU DEPRIVING YOUR BODY OF NUTRIENTS?

Your next step is to determine whether or not your daily habits are diminishing your vitamin and mineral supply. Many people do not realize the serious consequences that environmental forces, drugs, and their own daily habits can have in terms of nutritional deficiencies. Some factors, such as the air we breathe, are unavoidable, some can be controlled somewhat (medications and stress), and many are completely within our power to change (sugar, salt, and fat consumption). The ideal is to avoid as many of these poor habits as possible. If you are not ready to give up your favorite vice, then the least you can do is fortify the body so that your overall health will not be compromised.

Vitamin and Mineral Depleters

Food	Nutrient Depleted
caffeine	B complex, especially thiamine (B-1), inositol, potassium, zinc
alcohol	B complex, C, A, magnesium, zinc
sugar	B complex, chromium, zinc, manganese
high-fat/protein diet	calcium
refining process	B complex, many minerals
crash dieting	A, B complex, C, D, E, calcium, zinc, potassium
chlorinated water	E
inorganic iron	E
cigarettes	A, C, E, calcium, selenium
pollution	A, C, E, selenium
stress	B complex, C, zinc, all nutrients
infection	A, B complex, C, E, zinc
cooking	A, B complex, C
freezing	C, E
nitrites	A, C, E
estrogen	E, zinc, magnesium
aspirin	C, folic acid, pyridoxine (B-6)
antibiotics	B complex, C, K, potassium
antacids	thiamine (B-1), phosphorus
antihistamines	C
barbiturates	A, C, D, folic acid
cortisone	A, pyridoxine (B-6), C, D, zinc, potassium
Indocin	thiamine (B-1), C
laxatives/diuretics	A, D, E, K, potassium

How many of these items are a part of your life? Go ahead and circle them. What nutrients do you see you might be compromising? Do they appear more than once? Twice? Refer to your daily chart. Are you eating foods that supply these nutrients? For example, if you smoke, eat a lot of cooked and frozen foods, lunch meats, and bacon (high in nitrates), and take medications like aspirin or Indocin, you may require additional vitamin C. Keeping this in mind, check your chart again. How many foods do you eat that are high in vitamin C? If you are not eating fresh fruits and vegetables every day, you need to consider seriously adding them to your diet or taking vitamin C supplements.

Once you have thoroughly analyzed your dietary habits, both good and bad, you are ready to make some changes. Whatever you do, try not to tackle all your problems in the first week, or you will give up in frustration. The foods people choose to eat regularly often carry an enormous emotional force. Patterns of eating are related to many things—tradition, nurturing, and habit. Even to consider changing overnight is absurd. Because you *wish* to alter your habits doesn't mean that it is just going to happen; it will requirie determination and time.

There is no instant method for reversing a lifetime of faulty eating patterns. Remember that the slower you proceed, the greater your chances for success. Choose one area that you want to work on; when you feel that is under control, go for another, and then another.

You may not feel your body improve immediately, but after a few months, you should notice subtle changes: an increase in energy, less stomach distress, a clearer mind, more radiant skin and hair, stronger nails, easier and shorter menstrual periods, a sense of well-being, and a feeling of calmly energetic good health. I have experienced it, and I have seen it happen to many others. Believe me, a healthier diet and life-style will reward you in ways you cannot imagine.

READING YOUR BODY

Don't trash your new chart yet, even if you feel you have a handle on your daily eating patterns. There is a third column, remember? Symptoms. What are yours? Do you have a lot of those "normal" complaints? Are you run-down? Do you have the Monday morning droops? The afternoon slump? The blahs? Are you tired? List-less? Have "female problems"? Cramps? The premenstrual crazies? Read on.

Many people are suffering from marginal nutrient deficien-cies. They are not what you would call "sick"—that is, they don't have anything with a Latin-sounding name. You might just say they are "not up to par," "under the weather," or "out of sorts." A marginal deficiency is defined as a condition of gradual vitamin or mineral depletion in which there is evidence of lack of personal well-being associated with impaired physiological function.(1) Something is clearly out of sync, but tests normally do not reveal any major functional problem.

The body operates on a fresh and continuing supply of nutrients. When they are withheld for an extended period of time, functions deteriorate, setting off a series of reactions that begin subtly at the cellular level and gradually move up to the tissues and organs. Initially, the body compensates for deficiencies by using available nutrients. Not all nutrients, however, are stored for more than one day, and, in time, the stores of others get seriously low. Examples of these are the B vitamins and vitamin C.

Myron Brin, Ph.D., a nutrition researcher at Hoffman-La Roche (a pharmaceutical firm), and one of the pioneers in this area, has identified consecutive phases of marginal deficiencies in the body. In the preliminary stage, nutrients stored in the body's tissues are gradually depleted, because of low intake, poor absorp-tion, or abnormal metabolism. At this point, there are no symp-toms or detectable physical signs. As deficiencies progress to the biochemical stage (the stage at which changes can be detected through chemical tests) tissue stores are depleted. There are still no obvious clues, but silent destruction is occurring beneath the surface of the skin. Even though nothing can be detected on the outside, the tissue damage can have a significant effect on func-tions such as the body's ability to handle drugs, alcohol, or ex-posure to environmental chemicals properly, and on immunity to disease.(2)

Clues start appearing only in the final stage, where they show up as behavioral and psychological manifestations. Nonspecific symptoms such as loss of appetite, depression, anxiety, or insomnia may be among the first signals that you are undernourished. If you notice yourself writing these symptoms in several entries on your daily chart, you may consider it a warning of marginal nutrient deficiencies.

In the final stages, definite clinical signs are obvious and, if left untreated, eventually result in disease. Of course, this is what we want to avoid and, to a certain degree, can, by heeding our bodies' subtle, nonspecific signals before they reach a critical point.

Most bodily reactions involve several biochemical pathways or steps. Several nutrients, enzymes, and hormones may be required for one particular organ system to function. The lack of just one vitamin can easily result in a collection of different symptoms involving the skin, hair, eyes, mouth, or teeth, or the digestive, muscular, nervous, or reproductive systems. Adding to the confusion is the fact that the initial indications of many deficiencies are alarmingly similar—fatigue, weakness, minor aches and pains, headache, and so on.

Most researchers and practitioners in nutritional medicine agree, however, that certain physical clues point to specific nutrient deficiencies. For example, spoon-shaped fingernails with white spots, loss of the sense of smell or taste, and stretch marks are clinical signs of a zinc deficiency. These clues may be telling you that you are not taking in enough zinc, you have an increased need for the mineral, and/or you are not absorbing it.

Check Appendix B for a list of common physical signs and their associated nutrient deficiencies. While this list should not be used to make an exact diagnosis of your nutrient needs (other vitamins and minerals may also be involved) it gives the most common relationships and is a general reference guide to help you in establishing which nutrients you may need to supplement. Check to see if some of the signs apply to you, then circle the nutrients that correspond to the symptoms. Certain nutrients will probably appear more than once, indicating a likely deficiency. Before you run out and buy several bottles of vitamins, look at your diet. Are you eating foods that supply these nutrients? Are you engaging in habits that flush them out? Start here first to make needed changes.

Fine tuning your diet is something of a game, a continuous exercise, because your needs vary day to day, month to month, and season to season. As we move to a new stage of development, or into unusual circumstances (having an operation, going on the pill, fighting illness), we need to reevaluate and rebalance. What is correct for your body this month may not be true in five years. Being tuned in to the workings of our bodies becomes a constant challenge and, as our bodies respond to our care and attention, a constant reward.

Your Plan of Action
* Chart your dietary and life-style habits.
    * Check for nutrients taken in.
    * Check for nutrients depleted.
* Determine your symptoms.
* Determine your special circumstances.

If you are unsure of your nutrient status, you can use a systematic plan to determine which vitamins or minerals your diet may be lacking. Begin analyzing your diet and everyday habits by writing down what you routinely eat and drink. Then list all health habits that may cause nutrient depletion or poor absorption of nutrients (such as excess sugar, fat, coffee, alcohol, cigarette smoking). Lastly, list any recurring symptoms and special health problems and go over the lists in this section and Appendix B to see if you can make a connection between your symptoms and the symptoms of nutrient deficiencies. If you believe there is a possibility of a deficiency, look in Appendix C to see if you can get this nutrient in your daily diet. If you are not eating these foods, you will need to supplement.

Chapter 16

— ❧ —

Special Circumstances, Special Needs

From month to month, from birth to the giving of life to the change of life, women face a unique challenge to keep their body chemistry in balance.

—Richard Kunin, M.D.
Mega-Nutrition for Women

Women experience many dramatic physical transitions in their lives: They may become pregnant, nurse babies, take hormones, have hysterectomies, pass through menopause. Each of these conditions reflects alterations in hormonal balance that may necessitate special dietary reinforcement. The change may last only a short time, or it may extend into years. Being nutritionally prepared will ensure an easier transition both before and after the change, whether it is short or long term.

BIRTH CONTROL PILLS

In spite of all the risks associated with the pill (heart disease, blood clots, stroke, depression, liver disease), it is still the contraceptive method preferred by many young women. There is no guarantee that meganutrition can mitigate all of the above risks, but good eating habits and supplements can relieve the effect of malnutrition, which is the predisposing condition that eventually causes tissue irregularities and subsequent disease in many women who are taking oral contraceptives.

"One of the best-kept secrets about estrogen (and the same seems to be true of progestin) is that it wreaks havoc with nutrition—both vitamins and minerals," reveal the authors of *Women and the Crisis in Sex Hormones*, Barbara Seaman and Gideon Seaman, M.D.(1) Birth control pills lower body levels of the B vitamins: folic acid, pyridoxine (B-6), thiamine (B-1), riboflavin (B- 2), and cobalamin (B-12), as well as vitamins C and E, and the trace minerals zinc and magnesium. Certain other nutrients are increased: vitamin A, iron, and copper.

Pill users or women recovering from a long period of being on the pill need to make dietary changes to compensate for these nutritional imbalances. To restore the B-complex vitamins it is most important to stress foods high in B vitamins—whole grain breads, brown rice, leafy green vegetables, organ meats, and wheat germ—and to refrain from nonfoods that further decrease their supply, such as coffee, alcohol, and sugar.

The pill disturbs sugar metabolism, mildly in most women, but severely in up to 15 percent.(2) Generally speaking, the longer one takes the pill, the more pronounced the disturbance. For women who are taking hormones and also show several hypoglycemic symptoms, such as anxiety, dizziness, depression, lack of concentration, or crying spells, a diet that regulates blood-sugar levels is recommended. This means avoiding foods high in sugar and not going more than four hours without eating. Eating small meals of protein and complex carbohydrates every three to four hours is beneficial.

To reduce or overcome discomforts while taking hormones or to accelerate balancing the body chemistry after taking them, the following specific dietary supplements are recommended.

Nutritional Support for Women on the Pill

* B-complex supplying 10 mg each of thiamine (B-1), riboflavin (B-2), pyridoxine (B-6); 0.8 mg folic acid and 100 mcg cobalamin (B-12)

* additional 50 mg of B-6 (pyridoxine) for hypoglycemia, diabetes, depression

* vitamin C with bioflavenoids (45–500 mg)—higher doses if there are symptoms of bleeding gums, bruises, or spider veins on the arms or legs

* vitamin E (200–400 IU) with selenium (25 mcg)—take with meal in which fat is eaten or with lecithin tablet

* zinc (30–50 mg) 3 times per week

MENSTRUAL CRAMPS

Today, probably only the very ignorant, chauvinistic, or deeply threatened still believe that menstrual problems are imaginary or contrived. Both scientific understanding and human concern have brought us beyond that disgraceful attitude. The culprit causing the spasmlike pains that many women suffer is a substance called *prostaglandin.* When a woman experiences menstrual cramps accompanied by nausea, vomiting, diarrhea, fatigue, tension, and headaches, she is, more than likely, producing greater than normal amounts of this hormonelike chemical. The reason has not yet been determined; my own bias leads me to suspect that nutrition is involved.

Several researchers have found a strong correlation between hormone imbalances and vitamin and mineral deficiencies, and most menstrual problems seem to be caused by these hormonal imbalances. When the nutritional deficiency is corrected by diet and/or supplements, the hormone levels often return to normal.(3) This suggests that a lack of proper nutrients can result in a wide array of symptoms. For a more thorough explanation of the problem, I refer you to my other book, *Exclusively Female: A Nutrition Guide for Better Menstrual Health* (Hunter House, 1982).

Often, a simple change of diet to incorporate more complex

carbohydrates, fresh fruits and vegetables, and low fat proteins, while minimizing sugar, caffeine, and red meats, is enough to relieve monthly cramps. Many women have found that switching to a vegetable-based diet, especially the week before their periods, is equally beneficial. If this is not enough to relieve your cramps, supplement as follows:

Nutrients for Minimizing Cramps
* B Complex (10–30 mg)
* vitamin C (100–1000 mg)
* vitamin E (400 IU)
* calcium (1000–1500 mg)
* magnesium (500 mg)
* zinc (30–60 mg)
* L-tryptophan (1–2 gm)
* max EPA (3–10 g)

Do not forget exercise if you are bothered by cramps. Vigorous exercise four or five times a week on a regular basis can help prevent cramps. It forces deep breathing, which brings more oxygen to the blood, subsequently relaxing the uterus. Any aerobic exercise is good; fast-paced walking is all that some women need to reduce cramps.

PREMENSTRUAL SYNDROME

For years I refused to believe that my minor irritations and outbursts were in any way tied to my menstrual cycle. Headstrong quasi-feminist that I am, I believed that to admit to that possibility would mean that I was being controlled by my body. It took about fifteen years before I could accept this, and it wasn't my husband's reasonable discussions that altered my opinion, but my own research into the subject.

What I learned helped me recognize that my body was responsible for my moody behavior. I also discovered, first through research and then through experience, that my PMS symptoms were brought on or exacerbated by my own diet. I was living on coffee and sweets. For me, the amount of sugar and coffee I consumed were more reflective of my symptoms than the particular time of month. I was being controlled by my eating habits, not my hormones. Anytime I revert to my old life-style of coffee and cookies, I can recreate those exact PMS symptoms. There are those who would argue that I did not have a classic case of PMS, and maybe this is true. But many other women are on the fringe of PMS, so to speak, and can be helped as I was through dietary and supplemental assistance.

PMS is generating widespread interest among medical researchers and practitioners around the world. Clinics are cropping up, books are increasingly available, and new products are being formulated for the PMS woman. Doctors are experimenting with a variety of theories about the causes of PMS, from the hormonal, biochemical, and neuroendocrinal to the psychological and psychosocial. No one theory has been accepted totally. Possibilities include an excessive amount of estrogen, a deficiency of progesterone, an imbalance of prolactin, excessive amounts of prostaglandins, hormone allergy, decrease in endorphins, hypoglycemia, various vitamin and mineral deficiencies, abnormal metabolization of essential fatty acids, stress, and psychological factors. There are not enough scientific data to establish one theory clearly above all others. What clouds the issue is that no single treatment works for all women. Some women respond to progesterone therapy, some to dietary changes, and others to placebos.

This suggests that PMS is a condition involving a host of interacting factors. The treatment or treatments you require will depend on your particular circumstances. (The treatment you *get* will probably also depend on your doctor's prejudices.) Before hormonal therapy, you may want to try the safest and least invasive method: diet, nutritional supplements, and exercise. I cannot suggest that diet and exercise alone will work for every woman, but they may be the only remedy for some and they will at least help minimize symptoms in other women.

The connection between nutrient deficiencies and hormonal imbalances mentioned above works something like this: Without adequate nourishment our the endocrine glands cannot manufacture hormones in normal quantities. Nutritional deficiencies also lower the threshold to stress, increasing the hormonal imbalance.

Before I get ahead of myself, how can you be sure you have PMS? Even this point arouses controversy. The classic definition is that if you have one or several regular, recurring physical and psychological symptoms one or two weeks prior to menstruation, and these improve after the onset, you are a likely candidate. Katharina Dalton, a physician who has written extensively on the subject, emphasizes, "It is the absence of symptoms and the change of mood after menstruation back to being a happy, energetic, vivacious woman once more, which clinches the diagnosis."(4)

There are currently no definitive medical, hormonal, or psychological tests available in the United States for PMS. The diagnosis remains a subjective one, most likely made by the woman herself. Symptoms include irritability, mood swings, depression, hostility, confusion, coordination difficulties, fatigue, food binges, headaches, fainting, bloating, weight gain, constipation, acne, joint pain, and breast tenderness, to name but a few. In fact, more than 150 symptoms have been associated with premenstrual syndrome.

PMS appears to be more predominant in some women than others. It may follow

* any interruption of the normal menstrual cycle (after stopping birth control pills, after pregnancy, or after a lapse of periods);
* sterilization by tubal ligation or hysterectomy, and;
* pregnancy complicated by miscarriage or toxemia, or postpartum depression.

You are at an increased risk of having PMS if you have any of the following characteristics:

* You are over thirty.
* You are married.
* You have children.
* You do not exercise.
* You have difficulty maintaining your weight.

* There is significant emotional stress in your life.
* You have nutritional habits that include going long periods of time without eating and eating a lot of sugar, caffeine, and red meat.

Most experts agree that the best method for determining whether or not you have PMS is to keep a daily record of your symptoms for three months. You may use a calendar you have, design your own, or use one of the professional charts put out by various PMS authors and groups. I am partial to a little book called *Charting Your Way Thru PMS*, which not only offers a calendar but is filled with other information as well (see "Resources" for address). If you are using a home calendar, mark down the date your symptoms occur and when you menstruate. I suggest you also chart your food intake; this information will be a significant help in establishing necessary dietary changes.

Certain foods provoke and aggravate premenstrual symptoms; they should be eliminated a week or two before menstruation and minimized the rest of the month.

Red-Light Foods for PMS Sufferers

* Sugar, alcohol, caffeine, tea, and cigarettes: PMS women are often hypoglycemic, so a consistent blood-sugar level is important.
* Red meats: These are high in fat, which decreases the liver's efficiency in metabolizing hormones, and in phosphates, which use the body's calcium.
* Salt and high-sodium foods: These increase water retention and cause breast tenderness.
* Dairy products: These interfere with magnesium absorption and are high in sodium and fat.
* Cold foods and drinks: These can contribute to cramping by reducing abdominal circulation.

For the best results, reduce foods that aggravate PMS and increase foods that encourage relief of symptoms. Beneficial foods include complex carbohydrates, such as whole grains, vegetables, beans, rice, and fruits. Since fluid retention is widespread among women with menstrual problems, drinking about two quarts of water each day will help. Natural diuretics such as watermelon, strawberries, artichokes, asparagus, watercress, and parsley also help.

Many supplements designed specifically for the PMS woman can now be found in retail and health food stores. If you are taking multiple vitamins, check to see you are getting at least the minimum therapeutic doses of the following nutrients.

Nutrients and Their Potential Effects for the PMS Woman

Nutrient	*Effect*
B complex (10–30 mg)	regulates estrogen activity
vitamin B-6 (50–300 mg)	reduces water retention; calms nervous tension; preserves higher levels of magnesium
magnesium (500–2,000 mg)	normalizes glucose metabolism; produces calming effect
calcium (1,000–2,000 mg)	reduces pelvic pain, insomnia, bloating, nervousness
vitamin E (200–600 IU)	reduces breast pain and tenderness; normalizes production of sex hormones; is a mild prostaglandin inhibitor
vitamin C (500–1,000 mg)	reduces allergic response; relieves pain
lecithin (1 tsp)	helps prevent excessive fatty deposits in liver; deactivates estrogen
zinc (30–50 mg)	improves glucose tolerance; helps regulate prostaglandins
tryptophan (1–2 gm)	elevates serotonin level; lifts the spirits

Currently, a natural vegetable oil is receiving much publicity in PMS treatment. British studies have found that Evening Primrose Oil (EPO) relieved PMS in two-thirds of women who could not be helped by any other means; another 20 percent were greatly improved.(6) EPO has also been found useful in treating women with heavy and prolonged menstrual bleeding, and women suffering from fibrocystic breast disease.

Evening Primrose Oil is by far the richest source of gammalinoleic acid (GLA), one of the building blocks from which the body creates a specific prostaglandin (called PGE1). A deficiency of this one prostaglandin allows the hormone prolactin to become excessive in the body. Prolactin is another hormone found in greater than normal amounts in the PMS woman.

To be effective, EPO must be taken daily. The six to eight capsules, along with 50–200 mg of pyridoxine (vitamin B-6), should be divided into two or three doses during the day. Vitamin E (100–600 IU) plus the other nutrients involved in the biochemical conversion process are generally helpful. Always start slowly, with smaller doses, and increase as necessary. Remember, too, how slowly the body environment changes. Two to three months is not an unreasonable length of time to wait before noticing results.

Evening Primrose Oil is expensive, so I was pleased to read that Richard Kunin has found that the essential fatty acids in fish oils are just as effective in treating PMS. As little as 10 grams or 2 teaspoons of salmon oil a day can be effective.(7)

FIBROCYSTIC BREAST DISEASE

Fibrocystic breast disease (FBD), also called cystic mastitis, is the most common noncancerous breast condition among women. It is not a disease per se, but a growth of fibrous tissues that most frequently appears when a woman is in her late 30s or 40s and disappears with menopause. Fibrocystic breasts are uncomfortable, but the condition is not serious. Some 20 percent of the female population might, at some time in their lives, develop breast tenderness, swelling, discomfort, or noticeable lumps.

Breast cysts are influenced by the menstrual cycle and hormonal fluctuations, enlarging and becoming more painful just prior to the onset of the menstrual period. An imbalance in the estrogen/progesterone ratio seems to be responsible for both the cysts and the enlargement, but whether the important factor is the overproduction of estrogen or the underproduction of progesterone is not yet agreed upon by scientists.

Certain situations that result in a shifting hormonal balance may bring on FBD: It has been found in teenagers who have not achieved regular menstrual periods, women who have children late in life, women who have gained weight, women on estrogen treatment, and women under stress. Pregnancy and breastfeeding tend to improve the condition, as does menopause, unless, of course, estrogen hormone is taken.

Breast lumps are common and are usually a problem only because they are difficult to distinguish from cancerous lumps. If a lump fluctuates with your period, this usually indicates a harmless cyst. If you are past menopause, check the lump at the same time each month. (If you have FBD, you will still continue to have cystic changes in your breasts even though your periods have stopped.) If your lump does not move, have a gynecologist examine your breast.

There is no sure way to reduce breast lumps, but several dietary interventions have been found to work. Dr. John Minton, professor of clinical oncology at Ohio State University College of Medicine, found a connection between chemicals called methylxanthines and FBD. When a group of women with FBD abstained from coffee, tea, chocolate, soft drinks, and various drugs, all of which contain methylxanthines, 65 percent became free of breast lumps in one to six months.(8)

Since Dr. Minton's study, other researchers and clinicians have had similar success. Penny Budoff, M.D., conducted a test on herself and some of her patients who had premenstrual breast tenderness. They abstained from coffee and all felt that they had better months—less pain, less irritability, and milder cramps.(9)

Supplemental vitamin E, at levels of 400–800 IU per day, has been found effective in the treatment of breast tenderness. In a study where vitamin E was combined with reduced consumption of the xanthine compounds, evidence of improvement was found in 85 percent of the sample.(10) This should be good news for all "confirmed" coffee drinkers, who might take a little longer to give it up—but you should keep trying to give it up. Other dietary remedies for FBD that work for some women are to cut down on fat, salt, and cigarettes.

HIGH BLOOD PRESSURE

Elevated blood pressure, or *hypertension*, refers to a higher than normal force exerted by the blood against the elastic walls of the arteries. The heart generates pressure to pump blood throughout the body, and the muscular arteries contract to help it along. Each time the heart contracts, pressure in the arteries increases; each time the heart relaxes between beats, it drops; thus there is an upper (systolic) pressure and a lower (diastolic) pressure.

As a general rule, systolic pressure falls between 100 and 140 and diastolic pressure falls between 60 and 90. Many charts cite 120/80 as the optimum for a healthy adult, but remember, it is possible for you to have a different reading from the standard and still be normal and healthy. Several readings over a period of time will determine what is "normal" for you.

High blood pressure is a major health problem in the United States. According to the Department of Health and Human Services, it takes the lives of 250,000 Americans, or one in every eight adults, each year. When left untreated, high blood pressure can lead to heart disease, kidney disease, loss of vision, and stroke. Older adults, as well as other high-risk individuals, should have their blood pressure monitored regularly.

The most frightening thing about hypertension is that you might have an elevated blood pressure and still feel great. There are often no symptoms at all. It has been called the "silent killer" because roughly one-half of its victims don't know they have it.

According to the National Heart and Lung Institute, in a pamphlet titled "What Every Woman Should Know about High Blood Pressure," certain women fall into a higher risk category. Those women most susceptible include

* older women (high blood pressure incidents increases with age);
* women taking the pill (25 percent of all women who use oral contraceptives develop hypertension);(11)
* women near the end of pregnancy (hypertension usually subsides after the birth of the child); and
* nonwhite women (especially blacks).

Both men and women share increased risks related to life-style habits, especially smoking, overeating, chronic distress, and diets high in salt, fat, and sugar.

Even though high blood pressure is a high-risk factor for many diseases, such as heart disease, it is one of the easiest to treat. Good nutrition, exercise, weight control, and relaxation techniques can bring blood pressure down safely and effectively. This natural treatment is particularly desirable when you weigh it against the side effects of the common antihypertensive drugs (vasodilators, diuretics, and beta-blockers): depression, heart palpitations, dizziness, muscle spasms, menstrual irregularity, nausea, weakness, dry mouth, mental confusion, insomnia, headaches, drowsiness, nightmares, twitching, loss of sexual desire, rash, and swelling of the breasts, to name a few.

Women who have adverse reactions to drug therapy will be encouraged to know that the latest studies demonstrate that nutritional therapy may substitute for drugs in a sizable proportion of hypertensives or, if drugs are still needed, can lessen some unwanted biochemical side-effects of drug treatment.(12)

Weight reduction can bring elevated blood pressure to safer levels by lessening the work load on the circulatory system. In overweight individuals, the heart is forced to pump more blood through a more extensive system of blood vessels. It has been estimated that each extra pound of fat requires about a mile of capillaries to nourish it. Losing weight, therefore, should be one of the first measures in lowering blood pressure.

Decreasing chronic stress through relaxation techniques, deep breathing, yoga, and biofeedback is also being utilized more and more to combat high blood pressure. Emotionally disturbing situations that elicit the "fight or flight" response are characterized by increased heart rate, breathing, metabolism, and blood flow to the muscles, and increased blood pressure. According to Herbert Benson, M.D., author of *The Relaxation Response* and associate professor of medicine at the Harvard Medical School, repeated stimulation may lead from temporary to permanent elevation of blood pressure.(13)

Regular exercise can help to lower blood pressure by aiding weight control, minimizing stress, and directly influencing body metabolism and hormonal output. Dr. Robert Cade, professor of medicine at the University of Florida, has found that aerobic exercise caused a significant drop in blood pressure for 96 percent of the patients who tried it.(14) Regardless of any change in body weight, exercise has a beneficial effect on blood pressure.(15)

Even minimizing extraneous noises in your life can bring about a decrease in blood pressure. In a pamphlet published in 1972 by the U.S. Environmental Protection Agency on noise pollution, researchers explained the physiological responses to noise alone: "Blood vessels in the brain dilate while blood vessels in other parts of the body constrict. Blood pressure rises and the heart rhythm changes. The pupils of the eyes dilate. The blood cholesterol level rises. Various endocrine glands pour additional hormones into the blood. Even the stomach changes its rate of acid secretion. While most of these reactions are only temporary, the modern environment presents such ever-changing noise levels that some of the 'temporary' effects become chronic."

Loud or unexpected sounds (even moderate ones) act as stressful stimuli to the body. Many times a day, as we encounter barking dogs, telephones ringing, freeway traffic, noisy household appliances or machinery, television, radio, and rock music, the body prepares for "fight or flight" without being able to make an appropriate response. All this is repressed, or internalized, adding to prior chronic stress. If you can't eliminate the annoying disturbances in your environment, try exercise or relaxation techniques to help you avoid internalizing your stress.

What you eat, as well as what you do not eat, can cause or cure high blood pressure. A diet rich in nutrients emphasizing high-quality protein, fiber, and essential fatty acids has been found beneficial. Deemphasizing negative factors, such as salt, sugar, saturated fats, and cadmium, is equally vital.

Cadmium, a little understood trace element associated with environmental fumes, fertilizers, cigarette smoke, soft water, and highly refined foods, has been linked to high blood pressure. With age the body accumulates cadmium in the kidneys—up to 30,000 times the amount found in the body at birth.(16) In nature, cadmium exists balanced with zinc. When an imbalance occurs in the body, symptoms often follow. The amount of cadmium taken into the body seems to depend on the amount of zinc in the diet: The more zinc is available, the less cadmium is absorbed. The refining of food and environmental influences disturb the balance, leading to a buildup of the toxic mineral cadmium and a deficiency in the protective mineral zinc. When zinc is insufficient, as it is in many individuals, cadmium easily enters the system. Henry Schroeder, M.D., a world authority on the harmful effects of toxic minerals, believes that if we could remove cadmium from the blood vessels and replace it with zinc, regular drug treatment for high blood pressure could become unnecessary.(17)

Most people are aware of studies connecting salt intake to blood pressure. Researchers have identified tribes living in close physical proximity whose diets are similar in all respects except one—use of salt. Those who do use salt have markedly higher blood pressure readings than those who do not. The Japanese, who are known to consume 50 grams of salt a day, experience a common complication—the cause of half of all deaths in Japan is stroke.

Table salt is 40 percent sodium. One level teaspoon of table salt contains approximately 2,200 mg of pure sodium. Add common use of the saltshaker to a heavy diet of canned, cured, processed, and fast foods, and you can easily see why the average American's diet contains 10–15 grams of sodium each day (five to ten times what we require). The critical factor, however, may be the ratio of sodium to potassium. While a high amount of sodium is unhealthy, it is even worse when potassium is low. Richard Kunin, M.D., finds an elevated potassium level a better modifier of hypertension than elimination of salt.(18) Meat eaters, who tend to ingest more sodium in relation to potassium, tend to have higher blood pressure readings than vegetarians, whose diets reverse the ratio. A group of scientists in Israel, comparing the eating habits of vegetarians and meat eaters living close together and with the same genetic predisposition to hypertension, found that, though the vegetarians ate as much salt as their neighbors, they did not have high blood pressure. The researchers concluded that it was their potassium-rich diets that kept them safe.(19)

Potassium is abundant in many foods: Bananas, fresh vegetables, orange juice, beans, nuts, and molasses are the best sources. To maintain a high potassium level in the body, avoid eating processed foods or excessive amounts of meat, and when cooking, steam rather than boil to prevent loss. For those reluctant to abandon the saltshaker altogether, commercial salt substitutes that balance potassium and sodium will probably taste just as good.

There is a good deal of evidence that supplemental calcium (1,000 mg a day) can lower blood pressure in humans with mild hypertension.(20) Calcium, like potassium, causes the body to excrete more sodium. It also helps to regulate the contraction and relaxation of the blood vessels.

Magnesium interacts with calcium to lower blood pressure. Although the exact mechanism is not known, it has been suggested that magnesium regulates calcium entry into the muscular cells of the vascular system, where it can perform its relaxing effect. Because of their symbiotic relationship, it is important to take the two together.

Vitamins as well as minerals are instrumental in maintaining blood pressure levels. Needless to say, a healthy individual needs an adequate amount of all the nutrients.

A word of caution to those with severe hypertension: Since vitamin E can increase the strength of the heartbeat, it sometimes elevates blood pressure readings. Barbara Seaman and Gideon Seaman, M.D., recommend that those with high blood pressure, diabetes, or a rheumatic heart condition should take no more than 100–150 IU of vitamin E a day, and should introduce it gradually into the body in small doses.(21) It is best to consult your physician for specific instructions before supplementing.

Polyunsaturated oils, particularly the level of linoleic acid in the diet, play a role in regulating blood pressure. In countries where people consume more unsaturated than saturated fats, the incidence of high blood pressure is lower. In one study done in Finland of a group aged 40 to 50, even when salt intake was unchanged, blood pressure was significantly reduced by switching to a diet based on polyunsaturated oils.(22) It must be noted that when the group returned to their old eating habits, their higher blood pressure levels returned as well.

This indicates that substituting vegetable oils such as corn and safflower for animal fats is conducive to lower blood pressure. Recall, however, that there are two vegetable oils that are highly saturated and should not be eaten in large quantities: coconut and palm oils (see the section on fats in Chapter 13). These are often found in bakery and packaged products. Whole grains, legumes such as corn and soybeans, nuts, seeds, tuna, and salmon are rich in natural polyunsaturated oils.

Eating more onions and garlic has become a common practice for those trying to reduce their blood pressure. Both apparently contain a certain prostaglandin that appears to lower blood pressure. Clearly, some old wives' tales are based in fact.

The listing of vitamins and minerals below is not meant to be a recipe for lowering blood pressure; rather, it is intended to give you an appreciation for the many nutrients involved in this one regulating process. While individual nutrients help in specific ways, it is always the interaction among the nutrients that is most effective for total health.

Natural Treatment for Reducing High Blood Pressure

* Reduce intake of salt.
* Reduce intake of sugar, coffee, tea, and saturated fats.
* Reduce weight (if a problem).
* Eliminate smoking.
* Avoid oral contraceptives.
* Exercise.
* Learn how to deal with stress.
* Supplement daily with
    * calcium (1,000 mg),
    * magnesium (500 mg),
    * zinc (30 mg),
    * vitamin C (50–1,000 mg),
    * B-complex (10–20 mg), and
    * vitamin E (100–200 IU).
* Eat garlic (minced in foods or in capsule form).
* Eat polyunsaturated oils.

Chapter 17

———— ❧ ————

Exercise for Life

I don't bust my buns working out everyday for
nothing.

—Cher

USE IT OR LOSE IT

Exercise is as important to a healthy body as is good food. Preventing menopausal symptoms and the associated problems of aging involves more than what we do or do not eat. To be well prepared for midlife, we must engage in some form of physical exercise. "Virtually all the evidence we have points in the same direction," says Jack Wilmore, Ph.D., director of the Exercise and Sport Sciences Laboratory, University of Arizona. "Exercise makes you healthier and may impact longevity. It's time to become more aggressive in using exercise to improve overall health."(1)

Exercise literally can save your life; without it, your body deteriorates. There is no question that if you are inactive during your adult years, your bones will decalcify, leading to osteoporosis, the potentially fatal disease that is so prevalent among older women. Taking time out of your day to attend an exercise class, take a walk, or jog is not frivolous, it's essential.

If you want strong bones to support your frame and firm muscles to protect your internal organs when you reach 50, you should start your program early. But it is never too late to benefit from exercise; quite the contrary, with conditioning, you can have stronger muscles at 50 than you did at 30. I know I do, and I believe it was Jane Fonda who said that her body was in better condition at 49 than when she was 20. But optimum results come from planned preparation, not last-minute desperation.

Most people are aware of the role exercise plays in weight loss; if you are not, refer to Chapter 11. We are also familiar with its influence on the muscle-bone system. But there is more—much more—that exercise can do for your body, mind, and spirit. When you are working the entire body, the effects radiate throughout each and every organ, tissue, and cell. Consider the following list:

Benefits of Sustained, Regular Exercise

* When you exercise vigorously, you bring oxygen to every cell of the body, improving circulation, reducing fatigue, creating energy, and increasing your capacity for handling stress.

* Harvard studies show that aerobic exercise is a practical way to treat the emotional stress of daily living. It can reduce depression and give you a feeling of well-being.

* Regular exercise can prolong life, according to Dr. Ralph Passenbarger, Jr., of the Stanford University School of Medicine: "For each hour of physical activity, you can expect to live that hour over—and live one or two more hours to boot."(2)

* Physical activity stimulates digestion and increases the absorption of nutrients. A study performed by Dr. Gail Butterfield of the University of Southern California showed that active women had appreciably more vitamin C and iron in their blood-streams than did sedentary women.(3)

* Exercise helps you to sleep soundly.

* For women, exercise can help bring the hormones to a normal level, greatly reducing menstrual cramps, PMS, and hot flashes.

* Exercise helps the adrenal glands to convert andros-
  tenadione into estrone, the major source of estrogen
  after menopause, allowing for a smoother transition.
* Exercise is vital to weight control: It diminishes appetite, burns calories, builds muscle, and speeds up
  body metabolism.

Exercise comes in any number of forms. The kind that's best
for you depends on your age, level of fitness, and likes and dislikes.
Evaluate your goals before you buy shoes or equipment or sign up
at a health club. Make sure that what you choose is something you
want to pursue and can easily incorporate into your life. Your exercise program should not be approached like a fad diet—a temporary inconvenience you tolerate until you reach a desired goal.
To derive permanent benefits, you must continue a regular
program for the rest of your life. The kind of exercise you choose
today may change as you expand your goals and improve your level
of fitness, and you should keep adjusting and readjusting your
routines to accommodate your changing needs.

Women approaching menopause have specific fitness needs
that can best be met by engaging in three basic forms of exercise:
aerobic conditioning, muscle strengthening, and stretching. Within these groups, however, are endless variations; you can choose
the ones you like and that best fit into your daily schedule.

AEROBIC EXERCISE

The great thing about aerobic activity is that it can be completely individual, matched to your state of health. You don't have to
join an arduous dance class or run ten miles to get into shape. If
you are middle-aged, or even a young but unfit woman, simply
walking briskly will elevate your heart rate and give you the training effect you need.

The word *aerobic* simply means depending on oxygen
(which, of course, applies to all exercise). It is used by fitness
specialists to describe exercises that increase breathing and pulse
rates and produce predictable changes in the body (burning
calories, strengthening the cardiovascular system, toning the

muscles, and so on). All aerobic exercises have one thing in common: As your muscles work hard, they demand and use more oxygen. The main objective of an aerobic exercise program, according to "the father of aerobics," Kenneth Cooper, M.D., is to increase the maximum amount of oxygen that the body can process within a given time. This he calls aerobic capacity. It is dependent upon the ability to (i) rapidly breathe large amounts of air, (ii) forcefully deliver large volumes of blood, and (iii) effectively deliver oxygen to all parts of the body. Because it reflects the condition of the vital organs, aerobic capacity is often considered the best index of overall physical fitness.(4)

For your exercise workout to be aerobic, you must engage in continuous activity (not stop and start) that works the muscles and the heart for a period of 15–30 minutes at a specified intensity. This exercise must be practiced regularly; at least three times a week to maintain, five times to improve. The benefits of an aerobic workout are based on three factors: (i) It must be continuous, (ii) it must be regular, and (iii) it must be of a certain intensity. How hard you exercise is a personal decision that should be based on your heart rate. As intensity increases, oxygen demand goes up and your heart beats faster. The point is to keep within a specified range (training rate) during the conditioning period.

Before you begin exercising, it is important to determine the training rate that is right for you. You can do this by taking your pulse during the aerobic workout. If the exercise has truly been aerobic, your pulse will register between 60 and 80 percent of the maximum heart rate (MHR), which is around 220 beats a minute. The formula used to determine the training rate is based on this number, your age, and the percentage increase you want to achieve. The following example is for a person 45 years old.

MHR, 220–45 (age) = 175 x .60 (60%) = 105 beats a minute
    220–45   = 175 x .80   = 140 beats a minute

Therefore, the training range is 105 to 140 beats a minute.

The chart below will help you to select your target zone. As you can see, maximum heart rate drops with age, so you will need to make adjustments periodically.

Recommended Training Rate

Age	60%	70%	80%
20	120	140	160
30	114	133	152
40	108	126	146
50	102	119	140
60	96	112	128
70	90	105	120

Monitoring your pulse takes prior planning, especially if you do it on your own and are not a member of a class that includes pulse-taking as part of its program. If you have chosen to start walking briskly, jogging, or riding a stationary bike, for example, you need to prepare in advance. Remember two things: First, you will need a watch with a second hand; second, you must know in advance what your training rate should be. After you have been exercising for about five minutes, slow down just enough to focus on the second hand of your watch and take your pulse. Remember, do not stop your activity. Place your fingertips about an inch below your ear at the carotid artery and count the pulse beats for six seconds. (Do not use your thumb; it has a pulse of its own.) Add a zero to the number of beats you counted to get a per minute rate. If you are over your range, slow the pace down; if you are under, increase; if you are right on, continue exercising for the full 20–30 minutes. Eventually, you will feel instinctively what it is like to be within your range and you won't have to bother with this ritual.

There is a wide margin between the low-intensity training rate (60–70%) and the high-intensity training rate (70–80%)(Figure 10). What your rate should be depends on your fitness goals, age, and level of conditioning. To provide an explanation of the various ramifications of the two training rates, I interviewed Mary T. Lins, exercise physiologist at the Oaks at Ojai, a health resort in Southern California. The information that follows was gleaned from that interview.

When you exercise within the low-intensity range, your heartbeat is slower and you are not burning as many calories. However, in some cases this is just the effect you want, because the

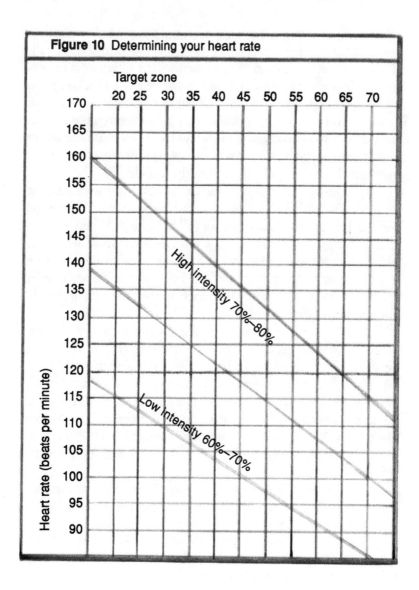

Figure 10 Determining your heart rate

calories you are burning are from fat only. Fat needs oxygen to burn, and at the lower rate more oxygen is taken in and is available for fat metabolization. As you increase the intensity of the exercise it becomes more difficult to breathe deeply, so less oxygen is inhaled. Less fat is burned, and the balance is stored as glycogen; however, you are burning more calories. So each range has its own reward: at low intensity, you burn fewer calories but more fat; at high intensity, you burn less fat but more calories, which come first from the glycogen supply, then from the muscle.

Either intensity provides your cardiovascular system with the same benefits, although you should double the amount of time you perform low-intensity exercises for full advantage. Whenever you reduce intensity, you must increase time. In other words, while one women may choose to jog for 20 minutes, another woman, who cannot jog or prefers not to, can get the same aerobic workout by walking briskly. The only difference is she must do it for 40 minutes rather than twenty.

Ms. Lins advises women who are just starting an aerobic exercise program, especially women over 40, to start at the lower range and work up gradually. If you join an aerobic dance or exercise class, it is best to begin with nonpercussive or low-impact movements, keeping one foot on the ground at all times while doing the exercises. You are not jumping, hopping, or running vigorously; you are mainly marching, prancing, and lifting your legs. Believe me, if exercise is new to you, this will definitely accelerate your pulse!

You can modify some percussive aerobic routines to suit your own level of fitness. Not all instructors are aware of or trained in body physiology, so if you are enrolled in a high-intensity percussive class, you may need to adapt the movements for yourself. It is important for you to be informed and alert to what is safe for your body; not all aerobics teachers are.

Even if you are strong, fit, and healthy, if you are over 40, there are certain exercises that could be harmful to you when done to excess. The mature woman needs to be careful not to do too many routines or repetitions that cause the full weight of the body to hit the floor all at once. When you land on both feet simultaneously, as opposed to alternating feet, damage can be caused to the reproductive system that may eventually result in fallen organs (uterus, bladder) or cause involuntary leakage.

Remember to keep your stomach tucked in during your aerobic workout to minimize stress to the internal organs. You will support the muscle fibers, lessen the momentum, and increase resistance. This also helps to tighten and tone the stomach and the lower back muscles.

Another precautionary measure that Ms. Lins emphasizes to avoid injuries is to pay attention to your bodily symptoms. Some fitness experts tend to stress charts and numbers and don't remind you that the body itself is the best barometer for determining the intensity of your workout. If you feel you are overexerting, if you are huffing and puffing so hard that you cannot talk, if you feel faint or notice a rush of fatigue, then, by all means, slow down. These symptoms could happen for any number of reasons: You could be out of condition, you could have a physical problem of which you are unaware, you could be coming down with an infection, you might be taking medication that is reacting to the energy output, and so on. Women going through menopause, particularly, may experience temperature changes brought on by exercise. Always listen to the wisdom of your body.

MUSCLE STRENGTHENING

The second kind of exercise women especially need is muscle strengthening. "If there is one area where women are neglectful," says Ms. Lins, "it is in developing their strength, especially in the upper body." The reason this has happened, she feels, is that women have feared becoming bulky and "masculine." Most of us now know this is an unreasonable fear, because we lack the male hormone, testosterone, that is primarily responsible for male musculature. Sometimes, if a woman has a high percentage of body fat (about 28 percent) and she starts a muscle-strenthening program before losing some of her fat, she may increase the muscle, so that, along with her body fat, the additional muscle may make her look bulky. I recommend that such women work first on losing through diet and aerobics, and then start a weight-training program.

There are numerous ways to strengthen individual muscle

groups. For the beginner, an aerobics class may help to strengthen certain muscles. Many exercises are designed to work the arms, legs, and abdomen. Floor exercises are especially good for this. Over a period of time these alone may not be enough to increase strength, because the body becomes accustomed to the same exercises and stays at a maintenance point. Then, one has to move up to weight resistance, using weights for floor exercises until that, too, becomes easy. Then it is time to proceed to heavier weights or machines. Whenever a program becomes easy, it is time to graduate to something a little less comfortable—that is, if you want to improve.

A weight-training program builds stamina, strength, and muscle tone, and is particularly instrumental in preventing loss of bone mass. Resistance causes stress to the body and, like aerobics, causes the production of more red blood cells, thereby strengthening the bone marrow. Weight training is more specific than aerobics in that you are working on one group of muscles. The effect carries through to the bone in that particular area of the body.

As you tone the upper body, you also reverse the pull of gravity that comes with increasing age. Many middle-aged women tend to get slightly bent over and have rounded shoulders. This can be avoided by concentrating on pulling back rather than giving in to the force. Weight training is useful in making you aware of your muscle groups and posture.

FLEXIBILITY

The third component of a well-rounded exercise program is flexibility. Muscles and connective tissue lose elasticity with disuse and age. Joints need to move through their full range of motion regularly to maintain flexibility. For many people, one simple form of exercise, stretching, will reduce joint pain and lower-back discomfort, improve posture, and minimize postexercise soreness.

There is a proper way to do everything—even stretching. Stretching should be slow and deliberate to be effective. Rapid or jerky movements are not beneficial and may even be harmful if there is too much tension placed on the muscle being stretched.

It is best to stretch your muscles when they are already warm.

So before you start stretching, exercise slowly in the same way you will be using your muscle. For example, warm up for running by jogging slowly, or warm up for tennis by swinging your racket. When you warm up, you raise the temperature of your muscles. This enables your muscles to contract more. Stretching before a vigorous workout reduces your chance of being injured, and stretching after a hard workout reduces muscle soreness and enhances muscle relaxation. After exercise, your muscles will gradually tighten with time, which will reduce your flexibility and increase your chances of injury. In summary, before each workout you should warm up and then stretch. After each workout, you should cool down and stretch again.

Stretching is the best way to increase your flexibility and to maintain a supple body. A good book to instruct you in various positions is Bob Anderson's *Stretching*. He makes the point that any stretch must be slow and sustained (a minimum of 20 seconds) to be effective.(5) Yoga, too, is excellent for improving flexibility.

THE BOTTOM LINE

Optimal fitness requires more than one kind of exercise. Mary Lins teaches that there are four major aspects to any fitness workout:

1. A warm-up is very important. You should not shock the body, especially at menopause when it is already coping with many other changes. Move your body gradually from a sedentary mode to an exercise mode. The object is to increase the body temperature, the heart rate, and the muscle demand slowly. Stretching and low-impact exercises, in which the feet stay on the floor, are good warm-up exercises.

2. Next comes the aerobic workout. This doesn't have to be a class, it can be any kind of aerobic activity; but the company helps. When you start on a brisk walk, don't forget that high-intensity aerobics must be done for a minimum of 15 minutes and 20 is better; low-intensity exercise should be sustained for a minimum of 40 minutes, and 60 is great.

3. After the aerobic session, when your muscles are warmed up, work on strengthening all the muscle groups. Don't just concentrate on your "problem" areas, include each and every muscle from your shoulders to your ankles. Mary Lins has devised strengthening exercises that are especially beneficial to women preparing for menopause. This eight-exercise program is illustrated and explained in Appendix F. (A handy booklet with these exercises can be ordered separately from the publisher.)

4. Cooling down is as essential as warming up. After a hard workout, you need to decrease your heart rate and body temperature gradually. Stretching will lengthen constricted muscles and help the body relieve itself of the toxins and lactic acid that have built up. Check your pulse rate again; according to exercise expert Covert Bailey, it is a more accurate measurement of health fitness than your weight.

As you become more physically fit, your resting pulse rate drops. Most women average around 78 to 84 beats per minute, while men average 72 to 78. Athletes occasionally drop as low as 35. My resting pulse rate was close to 100 beats per minute before I started exercising; now it is consistently 55. To get your true resting pulse rate, take it first thing in the morning before you get out of bed. Activity, drugs, coffee—almost anything can cause it to fluctuate. Count the beats for an entire minute; a six-second count such as you take during aerobics is not sufficient. You can also find an average resting pulse by taking it several times during the day. If it stays within a few beats per minute, you are close enough to have an adequate reading.

Remember, as you begin your exercise program, proceed slowly and cautiously. Don't become discouraged; it takes time before results are noticeable. And don't try to keep up with women who have taken dance classes since they could walk. Go at your own pace. Excellent guides for beginning aerobic programs are Dr. Kenneth Cooper's *The New Aerobics*, Covert Bailey's *Fit or Fat?*, and Sheila Cluff's *Aerobic Body Contouring*.

INTERVIEW: SHEILA CLUFF

For a clearer view on exercise principles important for women in general and midlife women in particular, I interviewed Sheila Cluff, a fitness expert in her middle years who owns and personally oversees two health spas, The Oaks at Ojai and The Palms at Palm Springs, California.

Linda: Middle-age spread is almost a cliché. Realistically, can women over 40 reshape their bodies? If so, how?

Sheila: To some extent we can, but it is very important that we accept our body type. There's no exercise program that will make a five-foot-one woman into a six-foot-two woman. Also, if you inherited a tendency to deposit fat on the hips rather than on the upper torso, an exercise program is not going to change that. We can't change our genetic type, but we can certainly develop more lean muscle mass; we can give more curves and more definition to the body; we can increase the size of the pectoral area, which will make the breasts look more attractive; we can reshape the arm so it doesn't have a lot of loose fat on it. I don't believe in spot reducing, but as we change our dietary patterns and our food planning, and, along with that, increase the muscle mass in the arm, we can reshape the arms just like we can reshape the legs and the abdominals. You can get to a certain point in changing your somatotype (body type), but after that you basically need to work with and realize you have inherited a particular body structure.

Linda: Many women hate the mere thought of exercising. What is the absolute minimum amount of exercise that a woman can do to maintain a moderate level of fitness?

Sheila: It depends on what that woman's goals are. Is it to be a champion tennis player, to achieve a higher level of energy, feel better, look better? Is it to maintain a level of fitness cardiovascularly; in other words, to prevent heart attacks? If that is her goal, she can cut her risk factors by getting out and walking briskly four times a week for 45 minutes, provided that other factors in her life, such as her cholesterol intake and sugar intake, are likewise controlled. This type of program will also help in developing a certain amount of strength in the lower extremities and the low hip area, but it will not be sufficient as far as the abdominals and the upper torso are concerned. So a woman must add to this a good 15 minutes of strengthening moves for the stomach and upper part of the body. She also needs to look at proper stretching. As a minimum, my feeling is that one hour, four times a week, combining the three elements of fitness: aerobic conditioning first (and, if you have to make a choice, make sure you do that even if you can't do the other things), strengthening the five major muscle groups in the body, and proper stretching.

Linda: Are there certain ages at which you should change your exercise program, especially the aerobics part, say, at 40, 50, or 60?

Sheila: I think you should change your aerobic conditioning program the way you change fashions. You don't really wear the same style at 40 that you wore at age 19. The body changes. You wear out. The bones become more brittle, although you can counteract that to a certain extent with exercise. So don't put stress on those joints through percussive aerobic conditioning when you have alternatives like swimming, riding a bicycle, and walking that are easier on the body at that age. You need to learn how to cut your risk factors as far as injuries are concerned at all ages, but most especially after the midlife years.

The main purpose of aerobic conditioning is to strengthen the most powerful muscle you have, your heart; to improve its stroke volume, which is the amount of blood the heart pumps out with each beat. You can do that in many different ways, so as you go through the different passages in life, simply alter the way you strengthen the heart. It may take you a little longer, as you grow older, but change your program to adjust to the changing body.

Linda: This is a personal question, but I think there are other women who probably want to know the answer, too. I've had so many people tell me that now that I'm over 40, I should no longer jog. But I've done it for 12 years and I can't imagine giving it up. Must I hang up my Nikes?

Sheila: Normally, I do not recommend jogging for a person over 40; it can be very stressful. If you've been a jogger all your life, if you have tested it enough and know that for your particular body type you seem to be able to tolerate it, and if you are doing it on a soft surface with good shoes, it's probably allright. Everything is a trade-off. All we can do is minimize risks.

Linda: What if you are over 40 and are planning to slow down, but when you go from a jogging program to a walking program you can't get your heart rate up to the training level?

Sheila: If you are in excellent condition, you have to increase the intensity of the walk and you can do that in two ways: One, you can carry small weights, and two, you can walk hills to increase the intensity. You can also walk longer.

Linda: For losing fat, is it better to exercise for a longer period of time at a slower pace or to have a shorter, faster workout?

Sheila: For losing fat you want low-intensity conditioning, in other words, 60 to 70 percent of your target or training zone. The time is not as important, although it has to be a minimum of 20 minutes. But it may take one person 2 minutes to get into her training zone, whereas it may take someone else who is in excellent condition 20 minutes at low intensity.

Linda: Is it good to alter your program with different kinds of exercises? For example, is it better to do aerobic dance one day and jog or ride a bike the next, or does it matter?

Sheila: There are two ways of approaching that. It is better for the body to alternate because obviously you work different muscle groups and that can be psychologically more pleasing to some people. Other people, of course, may like a steady routine. Whichever pleases you more emotionally becomes a motivator, and if you are motivated you are more likely to stay with your program. But there is no hard-and-fast rule.

Linda: Some women, like me, become overenthusiastic about exercising and want to do it every day. Is this good or should you take a day or two off a week and let your muscles rest?

Sheila: It depends on the intensity of the program. If you're on a sensible walking program, four or five miles a day, my feeling is that you can do that every day if you want to. If you're a jogger going six or seven miles, your body needs an opportunity to recoup, to get rid of the lactic acid. I do not believe in high-intensity workouts every single day; I would prefer you did it every second day. Light exercise as much as you want; real high-intensity exercise, give your body a chance to rest.

Linda: Is there anyone that should not exercise?

Sheila: You should not exercise when you have an infection, the flu, or a cold. Your body is fighting to get rid of the infection and you don't want to stress it in other ways. There are other precautions for certain people. Women with osteoporosis should not overstress the bones, which are already brittle. Water exercises would be better for them. People with back surgery must adjust their abdominal moves to compensate for that particular problem and find alternative exercises. Women in their last month of pregnancy would be better restricting their program to walking and stretching; they should not jump up and down. I believe there are exercises that certain people shouldn't do, but I don't believe there is anyone who shouldn't exercise.

Linda: Does a healthy woman need a fitness evaluation before she starts a sensible exercise program?

Sheila: Again, if you are over 40 and you plan to become heavily involved in an aerobic conditioning program, although you may have a perfectly normal resting pulse and be totally free from disease, there is always a slight risk that you may have inherited some type of heart problem that may not show up in the resting pulse. So, to be supercautious, it is always wise to have a stress EKG. To elevate your fitness level, you have to stress the muscles in the body and you have to do something to strengthen the power of the heart muscle; that could be potentially dangerous if there is something there of which you are not aware. But if you're simply deciding to go out and walk every day, and you're going to start with a couple of miles and gradually progress, I feel that you do not need a stress test. If it's going to be any more than that, I recommend it.

Linda: Do you have to hurt for your exercise to be effective? Do you have to "feel the burn"?

Sheila: There is a difference between the hurt and the burn. Never hurt in an exercise program. Nothing should be painful. The burn is really the body's signal that you are getting close to doing enough and the lactic acid is starting to build up in the muscle. A certain amount of that feeling is all right, but when it really becomes uncomfortable, the body is telling you to stop.

Linda: There seems to be a fine line, then, between the hurt and the burn. How can you tell when to stop?

Sheila: Stop if you feel direct pain. The burn or the feeling that you are really working your muscles to near capacity is a generalized fatigue. This is good. But if you feel a very specific discomfort in a localized area, that means you have gone beyond the burn, and should let up on that exercise.

There is a good way of knowing if you really have overdone it. If you feel extremely exhausted after your exercise class, you've done too much. If the next day you can barely get out of bed in the morning because your muscles are stiff and sore, you've definitely overworked. You should know the next day that you have exercised, but within a half hour after you have been moving about and your circulation has increased, the feeling should be gone. If you seriously hurt the next day, then you have pushed your body too fast too soon.

Linda: I think you have probably answered my next question. Why do so many women discontinue their exercise programs? Is it that they have done too much too soon?

Sheila: Yes, it's that New Year's resolution: "I'm going to get fit and skinny quick. I'm going to go on a diet. I'm going to the gym every day." Before you know it, you don't like the food you're eating, which in turn affects your mental attitude. You become depressed, crabby, or bitchy. You go to the gym. You do too much too soon. The next day you hurt. You feel wiped out and tired; you thought exercise was going to give you energy, instead, it's made you feel like you don't want to move. And you say, "Why am I doing all this? I thought I was going to feel better and now I feel worse."

Another common problem I see is that women often choose an exercise because a friend of theirs likes it, only to find out later that they don't. The only way you will continue a program is if you like it and if it fits easily into your daily schedule.

Linda: Can you give me some tips for the midlife woman in particular?

Sheila:

* If you are a beginner, know your fitness goal.
* Be realistic about the results you hope to achieve. A 50-year-old body is not going to be the same as a 20-year-old body, but it can be healthy, fit, and still look great.
* Become more body aware. Keep in mind the effects of gravity. Stand tall and maintain your posture throughout the day.
* Combine a good aerobic workout with muscle strengthening and stretching.
* Women especially need to emphasize their upper torso and abdominals. The older you get the more important this becomes.
* Don't think of body and facial massages as luxuries. They increase circulation and relax the entire body. That's a necessity.

Chapter 18

———— ❧ ————

Designing Your Supplement Program

Knowing is not enough; we must apply. Willing is not enough; we must do.

—Goethe

Preparing for menopause by eating the right foods and exercising is a great place to start, but it may not be enough to prevent menopausal symptoms or guard against bone loss. It is important that women consider the advantages of supplementation. The efficacy of vitamin supplements in treating a variety of symptoms has been proven. Nutritional remedies are no longer dismissed as old wives' tales. Controlled scientific studies and epidemiological surveys have validated many of the theories of nutrition researchers in the last few years.

Providing the body with a complete supply of vitamins, minerals, enzymes, amino acids, fatty acids, trace elements, and fluids is the surest safeguard against ill-functioning glands, hormonal disturbances, and physiological imbalances. It is simple logic: When the restorative and regenerative cycles in the body are completely supplied with the raw materials they need, the body has a better chance to maintain optimum functioning.

One thing cannot be emphasized enough: Supplements, even food-based vitamins and minerals, must not be substituted for healthy eating. Continuing to eat junk food while taking megadoses of vitamins is ridiculous—and probably dangerous. In fact, most supplements will not work in the context of an improper diet.

Supplements are best taken with food and with other nutrients. Vitamins and minerals rarely function independently. Whether any one nutrient is digested, absorbed, and properly utilized usually depends on the amount and availability of one or several other nutrients. If even one nutrient is missing, or in short supply, entire metabolic processes slow down or stop entirely. Some of the interdependent nutrients you should remember from this book are calcium and magnesium, iron and vitamin C, and calcium and vitamin D.

How much of each vitamin and mineral do you personally need? No book can tell you this; it depends on your diet history, your family history, and clinical symptoms. There is no predetermined amount of any nutrient that exactly fits each individual and each situation. The best that nutritionists and researchers can do is to provide guidelines, to indicate the different nutrients that have benefited most individuals under specific, monitored circumstances. It is up to you to determine how closely your condition matches these standards, and to judge when you may need more or less of a given nutrient, and when you need to revise your program. You know your body and your weaknesses better than anyone else. Based on the information already given you, you can analyze the data and work out your own program. Remember, if you are ever in doubt, or feel uneasy about the effects of your program, seek the guidance of a qualified nutritionist or consult your family doctor.

So, let's begin. The nucleus of any supplement program is generally the multiple vitamin/mineral formula. Many women will find that this is adequate to meet most of their needs. Appendix A lists vitamins and minerals and the dosage ranges generally recommended by nutritionists and clinicians. Even though some of the amounts go beyond RDA requirements, they are not considered unreasonable or excessive. When megadoses are called for, however, it is important to work with a physician. In large doses, any vitamin or mineral or other supplement acts as a drug, and must be carefully monitored. If you have any doubts or questions about vitamin and mineral safety, I recommend Patricia Hausman's *The Right Dose.*(1)

In addition to the basic formula outlined in Appendix A, further supplementation may be beneficial. If the multiple supplement you are taking doesn't contain an adequate amount of any nutrient (this is often true of calcium), or if you need a larger amount because of a specific problem (for example, vitamin E for breast pain), or if your daily habits are not going to change immediately (long-term smokers, drinkers, or coffee addicts), then it would be wise to add single nutrients.

Start to design your personal nutritional program by asking yourself the following questions:

* What diseases, weaknesses, and problems are common in my family?
* What is my diet like? (Take the time to review and complete your dietary chart as suggested in Chapter 15 if you haven't done so already.)
* What are my bad habits and what nutrients do they destroy?
* What are my symptoms? What nutrients are recommended?
* Can I get the nutrients I need in the amounts I need from food? Most of them? Some of them? Hardly any? (See Appendix C.)
* Are the amounts listed in my multiple supplement adequate for my needs?

So here, once again, are the steps to designing your nutrient supplement program: Once you have determined what nutrients you need, go first to Appendix C and see if you can get enough of that nutrient from the foods you eat. If not, buy a multiple vitamin and mineral supplement and see if that will eliminate the deficiency. For certain nutrients and special circumstances, more support may be indicated.

When you first begin your program, start slowly, adding one supplement at a time. This way, if you have an allergic reaction to a particular ingredient you will be able to determine the cause of the allergy. We are all susceptible to a variety of chemicals, both natural and synthetic; so, if one brand of a supplement produces unfavorable reactions, try another.

After a few months of a change in diet or supplementing you should begin to notice subtle changes in your hair, eyes, finger-nails, energy level, and sense of well-being. It is exciting to know that you really can control to a large extent how you feel and look by how well you nourish yourself and take care of your body.

I do not recommend or endorse any specific brand of vitamins. There are many excellent companies marketing their products through health food stores, mail order catalogs, and through direct marketing manufacturers.

There is much confusion concerning the relative virtues of natural versus synthetic products. The naturalists claim that their products, derived chiefly from plant sources, contain still uniden-tified "associated cofactors"; for example, natural vitamin C con-tains the entire C complex, which makes it that much more effective, whereas synthetic C is just ascorbic acid, nothing more. Those favoring synthetic products deny that there is any chemical difference, because in the test tube they all possess the same molecular properties. They also observe that, for people suffering from food allergies, the nonfood supplements are preferred. In general, nonfood supplements are cheaper. For what it's worth, I would like to share my own bias. Many clinicians I admire have found that natural vitamins are much less toxic when given in large amounts and they yield better results than the artificially produced varieties. So I generally recommend these.

Alan H. Nittler, M.D., insists on using natural nutrients to treat his patients. He explains the clinical difference between the two: "It is true that a sluggish organ, cell, or gland may be tem-porarily stimulated into action by large amounts of a separate syn-thetic factor, but if this is continued too long, it becomes similar to whipping a tired horse."(2) The prolonged action of synthetic nutrients is druglike; they overstimulate rather than nourish.

Once you start your program to to revamp your life and

promote health and well-being, don't expect miracles. Nutrients do not work like drugs. They act slowly to rebuild tissue and reestablish homeostasis. If it has taken your body years to create a hormonal imbalance, don't expect it to reverse in a few days. It may actually take a few months before you feel any noticeable changes. So be patient. Let the body mend in its own time. I must also mention that, as your body changes, you may actually feel worse for a few days before you feel better. This is normal, and you will find that the results are well worth the temporary transition.

The program that you are designing now is not engraved in stone. Your needs, like your life, are constantly changing. Some changes are short term (e.g., pregnancy), whereas others stay with us the rest of our lives. I continually readjust and fine tune my program as my life-style changes and my eating habits improve. And what I become more and more aware of is that the "purer" my daily intake—the less junk I put into my stomach—the less I need to supplement.

The real key to preparing for a healthy menopause—menopause without medicine—and a healthy second half of life is all-around good health: a nutritive diet, wise supplementation, regular physical exercise, and a positive mental attitude. Don't wait until you are going through the change to start thinking about your health. If you have prepared for the excitement and challenge of menopause far in advance of the midlife years, you will be ahead of the game, and your life will be the enjoyable, movable feast it was meant to be. Think about it, and start now.

APPENDIX A:
A Basic Nutrient Formula for Women

Nutrients	Range (RDA–Therapeutic)
Fat Soluble	
vitamin A	5000–20,000 IU
vitamin D	400–800 IU
vitamin E	25–800 IU
Water Soluble	
vitamin B-1 (thiamine)	1–30 mg
vitamin B-2 (riboflavin)	1.2–30 mg
vitamin B-3 (niacinamide)	13–50 mg
vitamin B-6 (pyridoxine)	2–200 mg
vitamin B-12 (cobalamin)	3–200 mcg
biotin*	150–500 mcg
folic acid	0.4–20 mg
pantothenic acid*	7–200 mg
PABA (para-aminobenzoic acid)*	20–50 mg
choline*	100–300 mg
inositol*	20–30 mg
vitamin C	60–2,000 mg
Minerals	
calcium	800–2000 mg
magnesium	300–800 mg
potassium*	1,875–5,625 mg
iodine (kelp)	150 mcg
iron	18–30 mg
zinc	15–30 mg
selenium	0.05–2 mg
manganese*	2.5–10 mg

chromium*	0.05–2 mg
copper*	2–3 mg
sodium*	1,100–3,300 mg

* No RDA established.

APPENDIX B:

Clinical Symptoms
of Nutrient Deficiencies

Ca—calcium	Cr—chromium
Cu—copper	EFA—essential fatty acids
Fe—iron	I—iodine
K—potassium	Mg—Magnesium
PABA—para-aminobenzoic acid	
Se—selenium	Zn—zinc

Body Area	Symptom	Possible Deficiency
Skin	dry, flaky	A, B, E, EFA
	oily	B-complex (especially B-6, choline, inositol)
	bruise easily	C, K
	wounds heal slowly	C, Zn
	yellow color	B-6, choline, Mg
	brown pigmentation	B, C, E
	prominent veins	C, bioflanvenoids, Zn
	pale, white	B, C, Fe
	stretch marks on hips, thighs, breasts	B, E, Zn
	backs of arms rough	A, digestion
Nails	brittle	Fe, Ca, protein, EFA
	white spots	Zn, Ca
	spoon-shaped	Fe, Zn, digestion
Eyes	dark circles underneath	B, K
	small yellow lumps on white part	A, E, Zn

Body Area	Symptom	Possible Deficiency
	night blindness, dry eyes	A
	red blood vessels around corners	general poor health
Hair	dull, dry	protein
	oily	choline, inositol
	hair splits and grows poorly	protein, Zn
	dermatitis	B, Zn, EFA
	hair thins out	B, protein, digestion, EFA
	dandruff	B
Mouth	canker sores	A, B-complex, Zn
	bad breath	B-complex (especially B-3), digestion
	cracks on corner of lips	B-1, B-2, B-3, digestion
Tongue	magenta coating	B-complex (especially B-12), K
	green cast	B-complex (especially B-6, choline)
	white	B-complex (especially choline), C
	thick white spots	A, B-complex
	scalloped sides	B-6, B-12, folic acid
Teeth and gums	bleeding and spongy gums	C, B-complex
	cavities	B-complex, Ca, Zn
	grinding teeth	Ca, Mg
	periodontal disease	Ca

Body Area	Symptom	Possible Deficiency
Gastro-intestinal system	enlarged liver	B-complex (especially choline, inositol), protein, lecithin
	nausea	A, B-3, B-6, Mg
	hemorrhoids	B-6, C, bioflavenoids, Mg
	bloating (gas)	B-complex, Zn, digestion
	hard bowel movement (infrequent)	Fe, fiber, digestion
Respiratory system	prone to infections	A, B-complex, C
	sinus	A, B-complex, C, K, Zn
	loss of sense of smell	A, B-complex, Zn
	dry membranes	A, D, E, Zn
Cardio-vascular system	increased heart rate	B-complex, C, E, Ca, Mg
	slow, irregular heartbeat	B-complex, K
	elevated blood pressure	Choline, Ca, K, Se, Cr
Muscular/skeletal	muscle weakness	B-complex, K
	muscle cramps	D, B-5, Ca, Mg
	stiff joints	B-complex, Ca, Mg
General	cold hands and feet	I
	loss of sense of taste	Zn
	insomnia	D, Ca, Mg
	varicose veins	C, E, Fe, Cu
	nervousness	B-complex (especially PABA), Ca, Mg
	low energy	B-complex, I, Fe
	poor memory	B-complex (especially inositol, choline), I, Mg

Body Area	Symptom	Possible Deficiency
	inability to recall dreams	B-6
	frequent ear wax	B-complex (especially choline, inositol), digestion

Sources: Jeffrey Bland, Ph.D., *Nutraerobics* (New York: Harper & Row, 1983); Richard A. Kunin, M.D., *Mega-Nutrition for Women* (New York: McGraw-Hill, 1983).

Appendix C:
Major Nutrient Guide

───────── ❧ ─────────

Vitamin A

3 oz. beef liver	43,390 IU
1/2 cup sweet potato, cooked	10,075
1/2 cantaloupe	9,240
1/2 cup pumpkin, cooked	3,800
2/3 cup broccoli, cooked	2,500
3/4 cup tomato juice	1,460

Other sources: carrots, squash, red peppers, spinach, eggs, peaches, swiss chard, endive, beet greens

Depleters: estrogen, heat, coffee, processed foods, low-fat diet

Vitamin D

1/4 lb. canned tuna/salmon	300 IU
1 cup whole milk	100
1/4 lb. beef liver	40
1 oz. butter	28
1 egg (yolk)	27

Other sources: fatty fish, organ meats, shrimp, fish liver oils, sun

Depleters: smog, mineral oil, cortisone, anticonvulsants

Vitamin E

1 cup raw filberts	13.5 IU
1 cup raw cucumber	12.6
1 cup raw kale	12.0
1 cup almonds	10.5
1 cup cole slaw	10.5
1 cup asparagus, cooked	3.9

Other sources: vegetable oils, sunflower seeds, whole-wheat breads, eggs, liver, collards, peanuts, wheat germ

Depleters: estrogen, mineral oil, chlorine, freezing, heat, oxygen, thyroid hormone, excess polyunsaturated oil

Vitamin B-1: Thiamine

2 tbsp brewer's yeast	3.00 mg
1 cup sunflower seeds	2.84
1 cup split peas, cooked	1.48
1 cup black beans	1.10
1 cup pecans	0.96
1/4 cup wheat germ, toasted	0.44
1 cup asparagus	0.24

Other sources: oatmeal, peanuts, liver, brown rice, fish

Depleters: heat, estrogen, stress, sulfa drugs, sugar, processed foods, smoking, alcohol, dieting, surgery, illness, coffee, tea

Vitamin B-2: Riboflavin

3 oz. beef liver	3.65 mg
1 cup brussels sprouts	2.00
1 cup almonds	1.31
3 tbsp. brewer's yeast	1.00
1 cup split peas, cooked	0.58
1 cup milk	0.34
1 cup broccoli, cooked	0.31

Other sources: organ meats, wheat cereals, burritos, red meats, yogurt, eggs, poultry, wheat germ, nuts, sesame seeds

Depleters: alcohol, antibiotics, estrogen, light, stress, junk foods, sulfa drugs, coffee, tea

Vitamin B-3: Niacin/Niacinamide

1 cup tuna (in water)	47.3 mg
3 oz. chicken (light meat)	10.0
1 cup broccoli	9.7
1 cup sunflower seeds	9.0

1 cup mushrooms	5.7
6 oz. haddock	5.4
21 tbsp. peanut butter	2.4

Other sources: pumpkin and squash seeds, cashews, un-creamed cottage cheese, split peas, beans, avocado, brewer's yeast

Depleters: sugar, antibiotics, alcohol, coffee, stress, estrogen, sulfa drugs, sleeping pills

Vitamin B-6: Pyridoxine

1 cup brown rice	1.00 mg
1 cup tuna (in water)	0.85
3 oz. beef liver	0.84
3 oz. chicken (white meat)	0.68
1 medium banana	0.76
1 cup fresh chestnuts	0.53

Other sources: sunflower seeds, alfalfa sprouts, wheat germ, fish, prunes, avocado, cabbage, grapes, green peas

Depleters: estrogen, cortisone, penicillin, heat, light, high protein diet, sugar, alcohol, stress, coffee

Folic Acid or Folacin

1 tbsp. brewer's yeast	313 mcg
1/2 cup black-eyed peas	230
1 cup orange juice	136
3 oz. beef liver	123
1 cup romaine lettuce	98
1/2 cantaloupe	82

Other sources: spinach, broccoli, beets, brussels sprouts, potatoes, almonds

Depleters: alcohol, stress, estrogen, heat, light, oxygen, sulfa drugs, sugar, caffeine

Pantothenic Acid

3 oz. beef liver	7.70 mg
1 cup mushrooms	2.70
1 cup sunflower seeds	2.00
1 cup wheat bran	1.60
1 egg	1.60
1 cup raw cabbage	1.30

Other sources: cashews, whole grains, wheat germ, salmon, beans, broccoli, peas

Depleters: heat, stress, methyl bromide, alcohol, sugar, coffee, smoking

Calcium

4 oz. sardines	496 mg
1 cup almonds	333
1 cup whole milk	298
1 cup yogurt (skim milk)	294
3 oz. salmon (with bones)	275
4 oz. tofu	154
1 cup broccoli	136

Other sources: cheese, corn tortillas, pinto beans, blackstrap molasses, sunflower seeds, chick-peas, kale

Depleters: antibiotics, smoking, high protein diets, sugar, fat, oxalic acid in spinach, inactivity

Potassium

1 medium papaya	710 mg
1/2 cantaloupe	682
1/2 cup butternut squash, cooked	600
1/2 cup lima beans	600
1 tbsp. blackstrap molasses	585
1/2 cup prunes	559
1 cup orange juice	496
watermelon (10 inch by 1 inch)	426

Other sources: spinach, pinto beans, halibut, banana, potato, sweet potato, green pepper, peach, apricot, tomato, soybeans

Depleters: diuretics, laxatives, malnutrition, fasting, surgery, estrogen, sugar, stress, coffee, alcohol

Magnesium

4 oz. tofu	126 mg
1/4 cup wheat germ	97
1/4 cup almonds	96
1/4 cup kidney beans, dried	75
1 cup shredded wheat	67
1 medium banana	58
1 cup oatmeal	50

Other sources: peanuts, potato, raw spinach, brown rice, peanut butter, salmon, milk, most nuts

Depleters: diuretics, alcohol, estrogen, phytic acid in whole grains, large amounts of zinc or fluoride

Iron

3 oz. beef liver	7.5 mg
1/2 cup wheat bran	7.2
1 cup pistachios	7.2
1/2 cup sunflower seeds	5.1
1 tbsp. blackstrap molasses	3.2
1/2 cup dried apricots	3.6
1/2 cup almonds	2.7
1/2 cup raisins	2.5
4 oz. tofu	2.5

Other sources: turkey, haddock, spinach, pumpkin seeds, cashews, lima beans, soybeans, peanuts, sprouts, peas, brewer's yeast

Depleters: estrogen, blood loss, high altitude, coffee, tea

Zinc

100 gm Pacific oysters	9.0 mg

1 cup raw Brazil nuts	7.1
1 cup cashews	6.1
3 oz. turkey (dark meat)	4.0
3 oz. turkey (light meat)	2.0
6 oz. white fish	2.0
1 tbsp. wheat germ	1.0

Other sources: red meat, almonds, lobster, whole grains, eggs, bran flakes, lentils, soybean sprouts

Depleters: infection, pernicious anemia, overactive thyroid, excess sweating, alcohol, diabetes, large amounts of vitamins B and C

APPENDIX D:
Natural Recipes for Hair Care

––––––––––––––––––– ❧ –––––––––––––––––––

In my quest for soft, manageable hair, I have found that natural products are equally as effective as store-bought concoctions, and at a fraction of the cost. Give a few a chance and see for yourself that they are as good—if not better.

* A hot-oil wrap once a month is great for dry, damaged hair. Take 1/2 cup of warm vegetable oil (safflower, sesame, corn, or olive) and add to it 1 tsp. of cider vinegar. Massage the mixture into your scalp and then wrap a hot towel around your head. When it has cooled down, repeat with more hot towels for two hours if you have the time. Even half and hour, I have found, is adequate for good results. Wash your hair two or three times to get rid of residue. Surprisingly, this oil wrap works better than many expensive conditioning creams I have tried.

* You can vary the oil wrap by using mayonnaise alone or with 2 tbsp. each of oil and honey. I'm not wild about the stickiness of honey, but others disagree.

* Egg shampoo is an indirect way of getting protein to the hair and scalp. It is far better if you eat the egg, thus feeding your hair follicles from within, but many individuals have found that applying the yolk to their hair softens it and makes it easier to manage. Beat the yolk in 1/2 cup of water and massage it in well. Keep it on for five to ten minutes and rinse with clear water.

* Stale beer adds protein to the hair in a similar fashion, as does 1/2 packet of unflavored gelatin in one cup of water.

* Plain yogurt provides protein and can eliminate dandruff. Leave on for 30 minutes before shampooing.

* Herbs will add brilliance to your hair. Brew herbs over low heat for 30 minutes to make the rinse. After shampooing, rinse your hair three times in the mixture. Carefully work the herbs into the scalp and do not wash with water between rinses. For light hair use camomile; for dark, sage.

* A very practical suggestion I learned at La Costa Health Resort is, when shampooing, massage your scalp vigorously with your fingertips or nails. Also, always rinse hair with cool water. It will make your hair shine and hold a set longer.

Appendix E:
Natural Home
Facial Treatments

───────────── ❧ ─────────────

Daily cleansing, toning, and moisturizing are imperative for the health of the skin at any age. The periodical removal of the dead outer layers of skin is important for all women, but even more so for older women or for women with chronic skin problems. Both weekly facial scrubs and masks can aid in sloughing off the useless dead cells and bacteria, allowing newly emerging healthy cells to take their place.

Facial Scrubs

* Vera Brown's favorite concoction is a combination of cornmeal (2 tsp.) and enough honey to provide a pastelike consistency. If the honey bothers you—it is very sticky—water can be substituted. Apply and massage gently. Remove with warm water and a terry washcloth.

* Emily Wilkens, a beauty expert who writes about the secrets from the super spas, has a variation of this recipe in her book, *More Secrets from the Super Spas*. She mixes equal quantities of cornmeal and regular oatmeal with hot water to make a paste. For extra cleansing and tightening, she suggests adding a few drops of camphor spirits to the rinse water. Don't rush to take it off; leave it on about 10 minutes.

Facial masks offer a variety of benefits. They can deep cleanse, tighten, and tone facial tissues. Whichever one you use, the procedure is the same: Clean your face thoroughly, apply the mask, and lie down with your feet elevated for about 20 minutes.

Remove the mask with a warm terry washcloth and follow your basic cleansing routine.

Masks for Normal to Dry Skin

* warm yogurt (can also be mixed with mashed avocado)
* whipped egg whites
* cornstarch, honey, milk (make a paste using equal amounts)
* crushed avocado
* papaya skin
* dried herbs from leftover teabags
* mashed banana (can also add honey)
* honey and egg whites in equal amounts (mix well)

Masks for Oily Skin or Oily Areas

* juice of 1 tomato, 1/2 lemon, 3 tsp. Fuller's Earth (available at pharmacies)
* 2 tsp. witch hazel, 1/2 tsp. yogurt, 3 tsp. Fuller's Earth
* 2 beaten egg whites, 1/4 tsp. baking soda, 1 drop spirits of camphor
* Vera Brown's favorite: contents of 10,000 IU capsule of vitamin A (sterilize a needle and puncture), the white of an egg, 1 tsp. sugar.

Natural Fresheners/Toners/Astringents

* Witch hazel has been used since time began, alone or with other ingredients such as cucumber juice or rose water. Mix equal portions and store in the refrigerator. Always rinse with cold water.
* Apple cider vinegar, too, can be used as is or combined with mint, lavender, or any blend of spices. Be sure to let it set for a few days before straining the herbs. Then boil with an equal amount of water, cool, and use.

* At the La Costa Health Resort in California, I learned about an effective astringent and skin normalizer. Simply pat buttermilk over the face and rinse with cold water.
* Vera Brown's favorite: Pure aloe vera (must be refrigerated).

APPENDIX F
Strengthening Exercises for Women from *The Oaks At Ojai* Spa

---------------------------- ૱ ----------------------------

These exercises are for muscle strengthening and have been specially designed to be of maximum benefit for menopausal women. Before you begin any exercise regimen, see your doctor for a complete physical, and review the exercises with him or her. If specific exercises, or a high level of exertion, are contraindicated, do not proceed except under supervision. Always stop if you experience ongoing pain or joint soreness. Remember, no amount of exercise is healthy if it is harming a specific part of your body.

The exercises are illustrated in two positions: A, the starting position, and B, the finishing position. Read the complete exercise before attempting it. Pay particular attention to the "don'ts" that are illustrated by the figures in the box.

Repetitions for all dumbbell movements: Two sets of fifteen repetitions for five pound weights. Fewer repetitions are required for heavier weights, more for lighter.

Cautions for all standing exercises: Keep back straight and knees slightly bent. Hold stomach muscles in. Keep breathing and control the movement.

Cautions for floor stomach exercises: Do not arch your back. Check with your hand to make sure your lower back touches the floor. Pull up with your stomach muscles and not with your neck. Control the movement at all times.

Exercise 1—Alternate Dumbbell Curl

Benefit: Tones the biceps and forearms.

Stand with torso straight and knees slightly bent. Hold a dumbbell in each hand with arms bent at the waist and palms facing upward. Keeping elbows close to each side, raise one weight while the other arm remains bent at the waist. Repeat this motion with the other arm and continue to alternate.

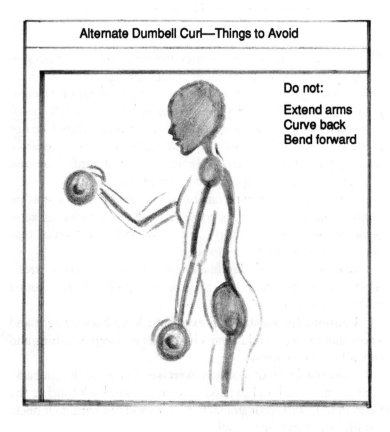

Alternate Dumbell Curl—Things to Avoid

Do not:

Extend arms
Curve back
Bend forward

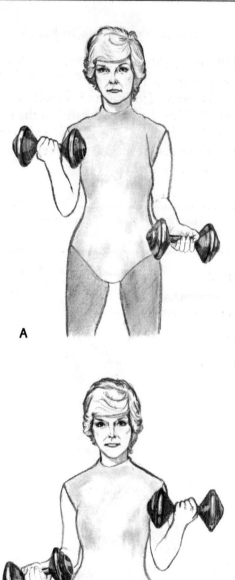

A

B

Exercise 2—Dumbbell Press

Benefit: Works all three sections of the shoulder muscles (deltoids), triceps, and upper chest.

Stand or sit erect. Hold one dumbbell in each hand at shoulder level. Weights should be parallel to the floor and palms facing forward. Press dumbbell slowly overhead as you exhale. Inhale and slowly lower dumbbell back to shoulder level. Repetitions are the same as for Exercise 1.

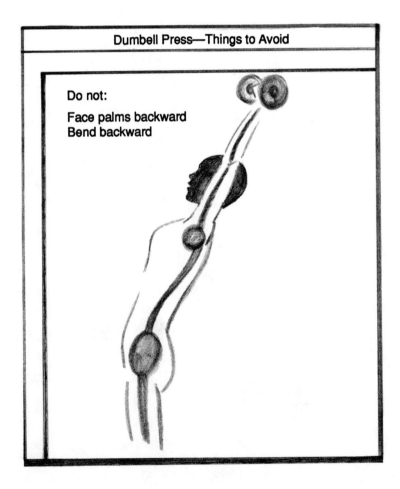

Dumbell Press—Things to Avoid

Do not:

Face palms backward
Bend backward

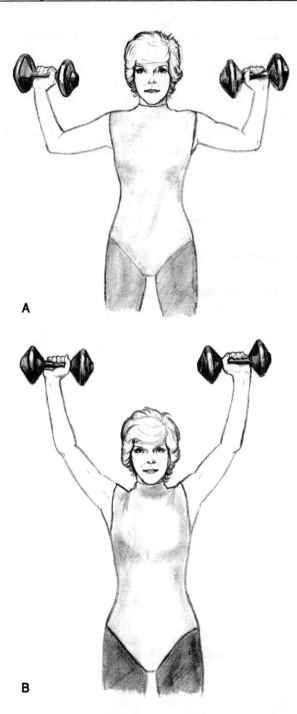

A

B

Exercise 3—Two-Arm Dumbbell Extension

Benefit: An all-around tricep developer.

Stand or sit, clasping one dumbbell with both hands, palms facing upward. Raise dumbbell above the head. Arms should be pulled all the way up so that the elbows are close to the ears. Inhale as you lower the dumbbell behind your head. Exhale as you raise the dumbbell over your head until elbows are nearly straight. Repetitions are the same as for Exercise 1.

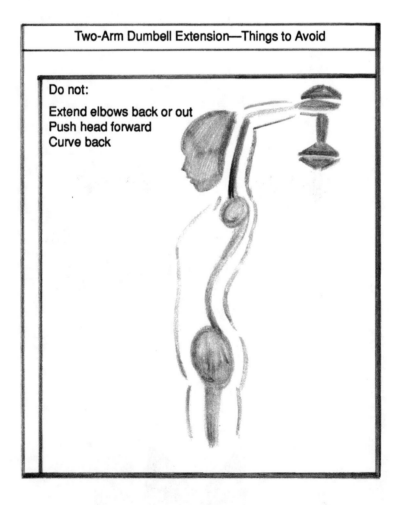

Two-Arm Dumbell Extension—Things to Avoid

Do not:

Extend elbows back or out
Push head forward
Curve back

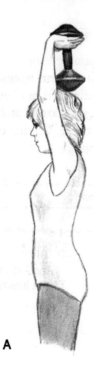

A

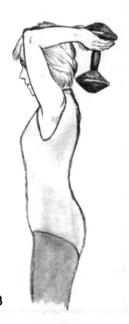

B

Exercise 4—Arm Pull

Benefit: An all-around shoulder and arm developer.

Stand with both knees and waist slightly bent, stomach and buttock muscles held firm. Hold arms directly in front of you. Pull back to the waist and then push arms straight. Extend and pull as many times as you can until your arms get tired. Wearing or holding weights makes the exercise more effective.

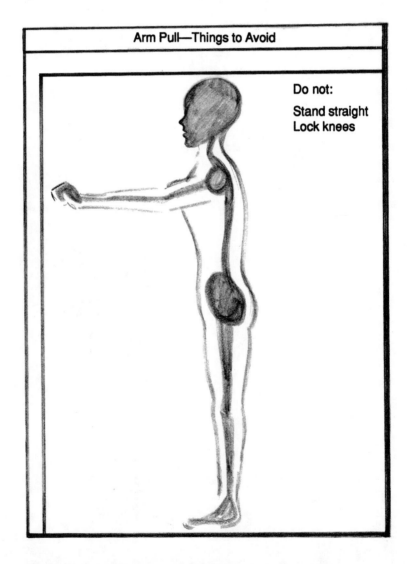

Arm Pull—Things to Avoid

Do not:

Stand straight
Lock knees

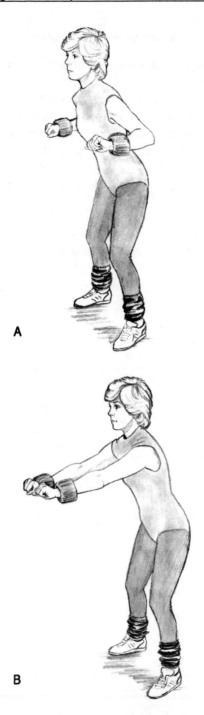

A

B

Exercise 5—Sit-up Crunch

Benefit: Strengthens abdominal muscles directly and back muscles indirectly.

Lie on the floor on back, with knees bent. With arms extended above chest, point hands toward the ceiling and look directly up. Raise upper torso, keeping stomach muscles tight and lower back pressed to the floor at all times. Be careful not to arch back. Exhale as you curl up, inhale as you release. Stay in control at all times. Go for twenty repetitions to start and add more as you are able.

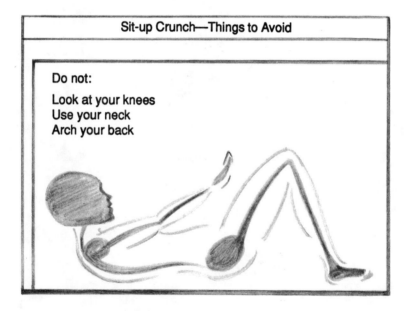

Sit-up Crunch—Things to Avoid

Do not:

Look at your knees
Use your neck
Arch your back

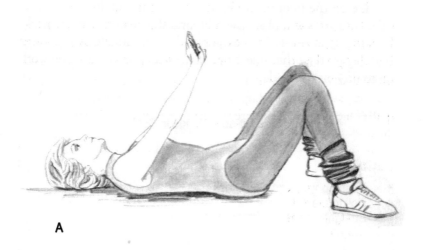

A

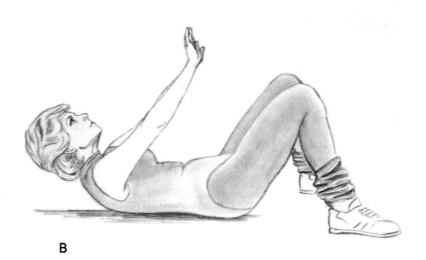

B

Exercise 6—Side Sit-up

Benefit: Strengthens the obliques (side stomach muscles).

Lie on the floor on back, with legs bent and dropped to one side. Fold arms and place them behind the head to support neck. Looking up at the ceiling, exhale and lift up. Inhale as you lower both legs to the other side. Start with twenty repetitions and work up to fifty on each side.

Side Sit-up—Things to Avoid

Do not:

Push up with arms and neck
Roll to the side
Straighten legs

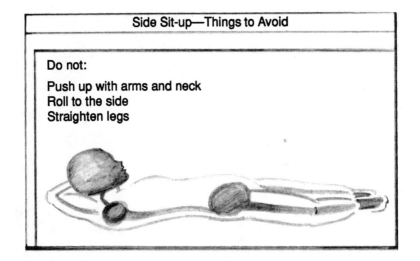

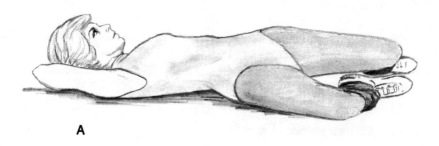

A

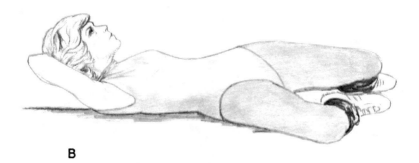

B

Exercise 7—Bicycle Twist

Benefit: Works the stomach, waist, shoulders, and upper thighs.

Lie on the floor on back, with arms clasped behind the head and legs straight. Lift both the left shoulder and the right knee off the floor simultaneously. Bring them as close together as is comfortably possible. Reverse arm and leg and continue cycling motion until tired.

Bicycle Twist—Things to Avoid

Do not:

Pull the neck sideways
Go past your comfort zone

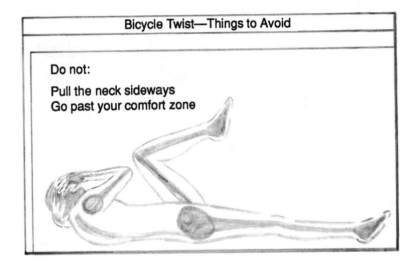

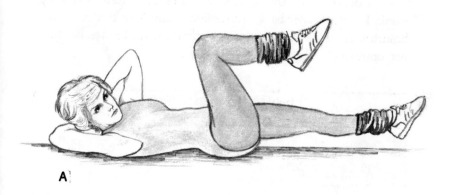

A

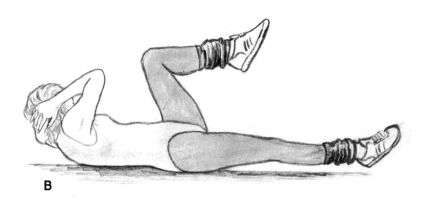

B

Exercise 8—Pelvic Tilt

Benefit: Strengthens and tones the stomach, buttocks, lower back, and internal organs. Also reverses the flow of blood and stimulates circulation.

Lie on the floor on back, with knees bent. Raise the lower trunk, keeping upper back on the floor. Raise four to five inches, hold, and then lower. Keep the buttocks tight at all times. Remember, do not raise too high. Do as many as you can.

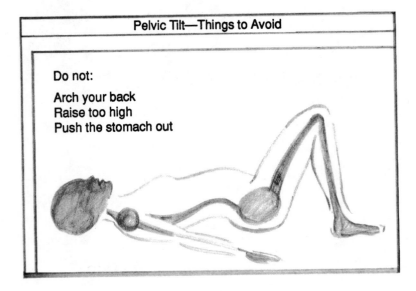

Pelvic Tilt—Things to Avoid

Do not:

Arch your back
Raise too high
Push the stomach out

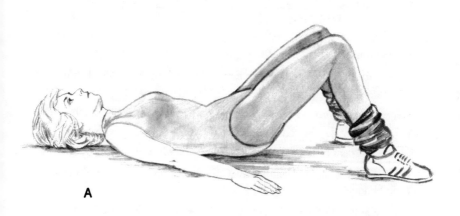

A

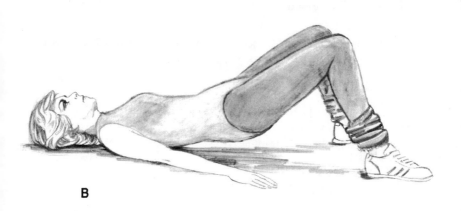

B

NOTES

———————————— ટૢ ————————————

Chapter 1

1. Robert A. Wilson, *Feminine Forever* (New York: M. Evans, 1966).

2. David R. Reuben, M.D., *Everything You Always Wanted to Know about Sex, but Were Afraid to Ask* (New York: Hawthorne Books, 1977), 292.

3. Sheldon H. Cherry, M.D., *For Women of All Ages: A Gynecologist's Guide to Modern Female Health Care* (New York: Macmillan, 1979), 205.

4. Boston Women's Health Book Collective, *Our Bodies, Ourselves* (New York: Simon & Schuster, 1971), 334.

5. Juanita Williams, *Psychology of Women* (New York: W. W. Norton, 1977), 360.

6. Cherry, *For Women of All Ages*, 205.

7. Barbara Evans, M.D., *Life Change: A Guide to the Menopause, Its Effects and Treatment* (London: Pan Books, 1979), 92.

8. Kaylan Pickford, *Always a Woman* (New York: Bantam Books, 1982).

9. Howard J. Osofsky, M.D., and Robert Seidenburg, M.D., "Is Female Menopausal Depression Inevitable?" *Obstetrics/Gynecology* 36 (October 1970): 611–14.

10. Napoleon Hill and W. Clement Stone, *Success Through a Positive Mental Attitude* (New York: Pocket Books, 1977), 7.

Chapter 2

1. R. J. Beard, ed., *The Menopause: A Guide to Current Research and Practice* (Lancaster, England: MTP Press, 1976), 30; Edmund R. Novak, M.D., Robert B. Greenblatt, M.D., and Herbert S. Kupperman, M.D., "Treating Menopausal Women—and Climacteric Men," *Medical World News* (July 28, 1974): 32–44.

2. Beard, *The Menopause*, 27.

3. Hershel Jick, Jane Porter, and Alan S. Morrison, "Relation Between Smoking and Age of Natural Menopause" (Report from the Boston Collaborative Drug Surveillance Program, Boston University Medical Center), *Lancet* 1 (June 25, 1977): 1354–55.

4. Louisa Rose, ed., *The Menopause Book* (New York: Hawthorne Books, Inc., 1977), 22.

5. Lila Nachtigall, M.D., with Joan Heilman, *The Lila Nachtigall Report* (New York: G. P. Putnam, 1977), 165.

6. Evans, *Life Change*, 38.

7. Rosetta Reitz, *Menopause: A Positive Approach* (Radnor, PA: Chilton, 1977), 19.

8. Louis Parish, M.D., *No Pause At All* (New York: Readers Digest Press, 1977), 30.

9. Winnifred Berg Cutler, Ph.D., Celso-Ramon Garcia, M.D., and David A. Edwards, Ph.D., *Menopause: A Guide for Women and the Men Who Love Them* (New York: W. W. Norton, 1983), 66.

10. Penny Wise Budoff, M.D., *No More Hot Flashes and Other Good News* (New York: G. P. Putnam, 1983), 19.

11. Beard, *The Menopause*, 46.

12. Howard L. Judd, M.D., "Menopause and Postmenopause," in Ralph C. Benson, M.D., *Current Obstetric and Gynecologic Diagnosis and Treatment*, 4th ed. (Los Altos, CA: Lange Medical Publications, 1982), 550.

13. Barbara Seaman and Gideon Seaman, M.D., *Women and the Crisis in Sex Hormones* (New York: Bantam Books, 1979), 365.

Chapter 3

1. Budoff, *No More Hot Flashes*, 37.

2. Reitz, *Menopause*, 27.

3. Niels H. Lauersen, M.D., and Eileen Stukane, *Listen to Your Body: A Gynecologist Answers Women's Most Intimate Questions* (New York: Berkley Books, 1983), 377.

4. John Yudkin, M.D., *Sweet and Dangerous* (New York: Bantam Books, 1973), 164.

5. Federation of Feminist Women's Health Centers, *A New View of a Woman's Body* (New York: Simon & Schuster, 1981), 96.

6. Seaman and Seaman, *Woman and the Crisis*, 472.

7. Michael Lesser, M.D., *Nutrition and Vitamin Therapy* (New York: Grove Press, 1980), 98.

8. Seaman and Seaman, *Women and the Crisis*, 445.

9. Sarah Harriman, *The Book of Ginseng* (New York: Jove, 1973), 25.

10. Robert C. Atkins, *Dr. Atkins' Nutrition Breakthrough: How to Treat Your Medical Condition Without Drugs* (New York: William Morrow, 1981), 131.

Chapter 4

1. Quentin R. Regestein, M.D., "Chronic Insomnia Provokes More Prescriptions than Diagnoses," *Journal of the American Medical Association* 237 (April 11, 1977): 1569.

2. Alan J. Cooper, "Tryptophan Antidepressant 'Physiological Sedative': Fact or Fancy?" *Psychopharmacology* 61 (1979): 97–102.

3. R. J. Wurtman, "Nutrients That Modify Brain Function," *Scientific American* (June 1982): 50–59.

4. Atkins, *Dr. Atkins' Nutrition Breakthrough*, 80.

5. Mark Brickland, *The Practical Encyclopedia of Natural Healing* (Emmaus, PA: Rodale Press, 1983), 311.

6. Emrika Padus, *The Woman's Encyclopedia of Health and Natural Healing* (Emmaus, PA: Rodale Press, 1981), 460.

Chapter 5

1. Barbara Edelstein, M.D., *The Woman Doctor's Medical Guide for Women* (New York: William Morrow, 1982), 82.

2. William Dufty, *Sugar Blues* (New York: Warner Books, 1975), 43.

3. R. O. Brennan, M.D., with William C. Mulligan, *Nutrigenetics: New Concepts for Relieving Hypoglycemia* (New York: Signet Books, 1977), 9.

4. Clement G. Martin, M.D., *Low Blood Sugar: The Hidden Menace of Hypoglycemia* (New York: Arco Publishing, 1981), 41.

5. Earl Mindell, *Earl Mindell's Vitamin Bible* (New York: Rawson, Wade, 1979), 176.

6. G. Collier and K. O'Dea, "Effect of Physical Form of Carbohydrate on the Postprandial Glucose, Insulin, and Gastric Inhibitory Polypeptide in Type 2 Diabetes," *American Journal of Clinical Nutrition* 36 (1982): 10.

7. T. Poynard and G. Tchobroutsky, "Pectin Efficacy in Insulin-Treated Diabetes," *Lancet* (January 18, 1980): 158.

8. Jeffrey Bland and Scott Rigden, *A Physician and Patient Survival Guide: Resource Guide Treating the Burnout Syndrome* (Gig Harbor, WA: Health

Communication, Inc., 1987), 87.

9. Brennan, *Nutrigenetics*, 160.

10. Richard A. Kunin, M.D., *Mega-Nutrition* (New York: McGraw-Hill, 1981), 125.

11. Broda Barnes, M.D., and Charlotte Barnes, *Hope for Hypoglycemia* (Fort Collins, CO: Robinson Press, 1978), 11.

12. Kunin, *Mega-Nutrition*, 86.

13. Georgia Witkin-Lanoil, Ph.D., *The Female Stress Syndrome: How to Recognize and Live with It* (New York: Newmarket Press, 1984).

Chapter 6

1. Morris Notelovitz, M.D., and Marsha Ware, *Stand Tall! The Informed Woman's Guide to Preventing Osteoporosis* (Gainesville, FL: Triad Publishing, 1982), 15.

2. Betty Kamen, Ph.D., and Si Kamen, *Osteoporosis: What It Is, How to Prevent It, How to Stop It* (New York: Pinnacle Books, 1984), 7.

3. Notelovitz and Ware, *Stand Tall!*, 40.

4. Judd, "Menopause and Postmenopause," 554.

5. Kamen and Kaman, *Osteoporosis* , 97.

6. Council on Scientific Affairs, American Medical Association, "Estrogen Replacement in the Menopause," *Journal of the American Medical Association* 249 (1983): 359–61.

7. Boston Women's Health Book Collective, *Our Bodies, Ourselves*, 332.

8. Barbara S. Hulka, M.D., Lloyd E. Chambles, Ph.D., David Kaufman, M.D., Wesley C. Fowler, Jr., M.D., Bernard G. Greenberg, Ph.D., "Protection Against Endometrial Carcinoma by Combination-Product Oral Contraceptives," *Journal of the American Medical Association* 247 (1982): 475-77.

9. R. W. Smith, W. R. Eyler, and R. C. Mellinger, "On the Incidence of Senile Osteoporosis," *Annals of Internal Medicine* 52 (1960): 773–76.

10. Jeffrey Bland, Ph.D., *Nutraerobics* (New York: Harper & Row, 1983), 256.

11. Notelovitz and Ware, *Stand Tall!*, 72.

12. John F. Aloia, M.D., et al., "Prevention of Involutional Bone Loss by Exercise," *Annals of Internal Medicine* 89 (1978): 356–58.

Chapter 7

1. Jane Fonda, with Mignon McCarthy, *Women Coming of Age* (New York: Simon & Schuster, 1984), 60.

2. Padus, *The Woman's Encyclopedia*, 271.

3. Richard A. Kunin, M.D., *Mega-Nutrition for Women* (New York: McGraw-Hill, 1983), 46.

Chapter 8

1. Shere Hite, *The Hite Report: A Nationwide Study of Female Sexuality* (New York: Dell, 1981), 508.

2. Linda Madaras, Jane Patterson, and Peter Schlick, *Womancare: Gynecological Guide to Your Body* (New York: Avon, 1981), 611.

3. Lauersen and Stukane, *Listen to Your Body*, 386.

4. Vidal S. Clay, *Women: Menopause and Middle Age* (Pittsburgh, PA: Know, 1977), 92.

5. Durk Pearson and Sandy Shaw, *Life Extension: A Practical Scientific Approach* (New York: Warner Books, 1982), 205.

6. Bland, *Nutraerobics*, 17.

Chapter 9

1. Edelstein, *The Woman Doctor's Medical Guide*, 132.

2. Lillian B. Rubin, *Women of a Certain Age: The Midlife Search for Self* (New York: Harper & Row, 1979), 54.

3. Pauline Bart, "Depression in Middle-Aged Women," in Vivian Gornick and Barbara K. Moran, eds., *Woman in Sexist Society: Studies in Power and Powerlessness* (New York: Basic Books, 1971), 110.

4. Sadja Greenwood, M.D., *Menopause Naturally: Preparing for the Second Half of Life* (San Francisco: Volcano Press, 1984), 73.

5. E. Cheraskin, M.D., and W. M. Ringdorf, Jr., with Arline Brecher, *Psychodietetics: Food as the Key to Emotional Health* (New York: Bantam Books, 1981), 226.

6. Roger J. Williams, Ph.D., *Nutrition in a Nutshell* (Garden City, NY: Doubleday, 1962), 94.

7. Alan J. Gelenberg, M.D., et al., "Tyrosine for the Treatment of Depression," *American Journal of Psychiatry* 137 (May 1980): 622.

8. Cheraskin and Ringdorf, *Psychodietetics*, 72.

9. *American Health* (March/April, 1984): 28.

Chapter 10

1. "Stress: Can We Cope?" *Time* (June 6, 1983): 48–54.

2. Colette Dowling, *The Cinderella Complex* (New York: Pocket Books, 1981), 201.

3. Nora Scott Kinzer, *Stress and the American Woman* (New York: Ballantine Books, 1979), 107.

4. Witkin-Lanoil, *The Female Stress Syndrome*, 71.

5. David Ward Tresmer, *Fear of Success* (New York: Plenum Press, 1977).

6. Dowling, *The Cinderella Complex*, 193.

7. *Orange County Register* (March 11, 1985): D-1.

8. Carl Pfeiffer, M.D., *Mental and Elemental Nutrients: A Physician's Guide to Nutrition and Health Care* (New Canaan, CT: Keats Publishing, 1975), 172.

Chapter 11

1. Cheraskin and Ringdorf, *Psychodietetics*, 30.

2. Edelstein, *The Woman Doctor's Medical Guide*, 146.

Chapter 12

1. Henry Beiler, *Food Is Your Best Medicine* (New York: Random House, 1965), 34.

2. R. S. Murphy and G. A. Muhad, "Methodologic Considerations of the National Health and Nutrition Examination Survey," *American Journal of Clinical Nutrition* (Suppl.) 35 (May 1982).

3. Ibid.

4. U.S. Department of Health and Human Services, *Ten Leading Causes of Death in the U.S., 1977* (Washington, DC: Government Printing Office, 1980).

5. Select Committee on Nutrition and Human Needs, U.S. Senate, *Dietary Goals for the United States* (Washington, DC: Government Printing Office, 1977).

6. Sherwood L. Gorbach, M.D., David R. Zimmerman, and Margo Woods, *The Doctor's Anti-Breast Cancer Diet* (New York: Simon & Schuster,

1984), 15.

7. Weston Price, *Nutrition and Physical Degeneration* (Santa Monica, CA: Price-Potter Foundation, 1970).

8. Kunin, *Mega-Nutrition for Women*, 12.

Chapter 13

1. Frances Moore Lappe, *Diet for a Small Planet* (New York: Ballantine Books, 1982).

Chapter 14

1. Carlton Fredericks, *Program for Living Longer* (New York: Simon & Schuster, 1983), 30.

2. Lauersen and Stukane, *Listen to Your Body*, 120.

3. Peter W. Curatolo, M.D., and David Robertson, M.D., "The Health Consequences of Caffeine," *Annals of Internal Medicine* 98 (1983): 641–53.

4. Lynn Rosenberg et al., "Breast Cancer and Alcoholic Beverage Consumption," *Lancet* (January 30, 1982): 267–69.

5. Bland, *Nutraerobics*, 214.

Chapter 15

1. Bland, *Nutraerobics*, 68.

2. *American Journal of Clinical Nutrition* 24 (1971): 269.

Chapter 16

1. Seaman and Seaman, *Women and the Crisis*, 135.

2. Ibid., 161.

3. Newbold, *Mega-Nutrients for Your Nerves* (New York: Berkely Publishing Co., 1975), 213.

4. Katharina Dalton, M.D., *Once a Month* (Claremont, CA: Hunter House, 1987), 13.

5. Janet Hopson and Anne Rosenfield, "PMS: Puzzling Monthly Symptoms," *Psychology Today* (August 1984): 30–38.

6. Richard Passwater, *Evening Primrose Oil* (New Canaan, CT: Keats Publishing, 1981), 22.

7. Kunin, *Mega-Nutrition for Women*, 76.

8. J. Minton, Webster Foecking, et al. "Response of Fibrocystic Breast Disease to Caffeine Withdrawal and Correlation of Cyclic Nucleotides with Breast Disease," *American Journal of Obstetrics and Gynecology* 135 (1979): 157.

9. Penny Wise Budoff, *No More Menstrual Cramps and Other Good News* (New York: G. P. Putnam, 1981), 73.

10. P. M. Farrell and J. G. Bieri, "Megavitamin E Supplementation in Man," *American Journal of Clinical Nutrition* 28 (1975): 1381.

11. Boston Women's Health Book Collective, *The New Our Bodies, Ourselves* (New York: Simon & Schuster, 1984), 541.

12. R. Stamler et al., "Nutrition Therapy for High Blood Pressure: Final Report of a Four-Year Randomized Controlled Trial—the Hypertension Control Program," *Journal of the American Medical Association* 257 (March 20, 1987): 1484.

13. Herbert Benson, M.D., *The Mind/Body Effect: How Behavioral Medicine Can Show You the Way to Better Health* (New York: Berkley Books, 1981), 98.

14. Mindell, *Earl Mindell's Pill Bible*, 267.

15. M. Krotkiewski et al., "Effects of Long-Term Physical Training on Body Fat, Metabolism, and Blood Pressure in Obesity," *Metabolism* 28 (1979): 650–58.

16. Lesser, *Nutrition and Vitamin Therapy*, 156.

17. Henry Schroeder, M.D., *The Poisons Around Us* (New Canaan, CT: Keats Publishing, 1974), 86.

18. Kunin, *Mega-Nutrition for Women*, 84.

19. Orna Ophir, M.D., et al., "Low Blood Pressure in Vegetarians: The Possible Role of Potassium," *American Journal of Clinical Nutrition* 37 (1983): 755–62.

20. D. A. McCarron and C. D. Morris, "Blood Pressure Response to Oral Calcium in Mild to Moderate Hypertension: A Randomized, Double-Blind, Placebo-Controlled, Crossover Trial," *Annals of Internal Medicine* 103 (1985): 825.

21. Seaman and Seaman, *Women and the Crisis*, 445.

22. James Iacono et al., "Effect of Dietary Fat on Blood Pressure in a Rural Finnish Population," *American Journal of Clinical Nutrition* 38 (December 1983): 860–69.

Chapter 17

1. Sharie Miller, "Getting Started, Staying Fit," *Vogue* 175 (April 1985): 340.

2. Philip Elmer-Dewitt, "Extra Years for Extra Effort," *Time* (March 17, 1986): 66.

3. Kunin, *Mega-Nutrition*, 150.

4. Kenneth H. Cooper, M.D., *The New Aerobics* (New York: Bantam Books, 1981), 16.

5. Bob Anderson, *Stretching* (Bolinas, CA: Shelter Publications, 1980).

Chapter 18

1. Patricia Hausman, M.S., *The Right Dose: How to Take Vitamins and Minerals Safely* (Emmaus, PA: Rodale Press, 1987).

2. Alan H. Nittler, M.D., *A New Breed of Doctor* (New York: Pyramid House, 1972), 49.

Glossary

———————— ❧ ————————

Adipose—(fat) commonly used in describing the part of the body where fat is stored.

Adrenal glands—small, pyramid-shaped glands situated on top of each kidney that secrete various substances, among which are the steroid hormones androgen, estrogen, and progestogen.

Adrenal cortex—outer part of the adrenal gland that secretes cortisone-like hormones.

Adrenaline—neurotransmitter produced by the adrenal gland, released in response to fear, heightened emotion, or physiological stress.

Amenorrhea—failure to menstruate.

Amino acid—organic compound of carbon, hydrogen, oxygen, and nitrogen; the "building blocks" of protein.

Amphetamine—drug used as a stimulant for people in tired or depressed states and also to decrease nasal congestion and to decrease appetite.

Androstenedione—weak androgen abundantly secreted by menopausal ovaries as well as the adrenal glands; a major source of estrogen during and after menopause.

Anovulatory cycle—menstrual cycle without ovulation or the release of an egg.

Antihypertensive—medication used to lower high blood pressure.

Antioxidant—substance that prevents oxidation or inhibits reactions promoted by oxygen.

Atrophy—withering of an organ that had previously been normally developed.

Basal metabolic rate (BMR)—temperature of the body at the time of awakening each morning.

Bioflavenoid—constituent of the vitamin C complex.

Blood-sugar control mechanism—regulates the amount of sugar in the bloodstream; includes the pancreas, insulin, glucagon, and adrenaline.

Blood-sugar level—amount of glucose (sugar) circulating in the bloodstream (normal levels are between 80 and 120 milligrams).

Calcitonin—"calcium-sparing" hormone released primarily by the thyroid gland; acts to slow down the breakdown of bone.

Calcium balance—net processes in which calcium enters the body (through the diet) and leaves the body (through sweat, urine, and feces).

Carotene—compound in plants that the body converts into vitamin A.

Carotid arteries—large arteries on either side of the neck that supply blood to the head.

Catecholamines—breakdown products of adrenaline.

Cellulose—carbohydrate found in the woody part of plants and trees; provides fiber to the body.

Cervix—narrow lower end of the uterus that extends into the vagina.

Chelation—process of covering a mineral with an amino acid to enhance its absorption rate.

Collagen—protein that is the supportive component of bone, connective tissue, cartilage, and skin.

Corpus luteum—"yellow body" seen in the ovary after ovulation, the cells of which produce progesterone and estrogen as well as other hormones.

Corticosteriods—drugs that resemble the adrenal hormones.

Cortisone—adrenal hormone that can be harmful to bones; also a drug that resembles the adrenal hormone.

Cross-linking—oxidation reaction in which undesirable bonds form between nucleic acids (RNA and DNA), between proteins (often as links between sulfur atoms), between lipids, or any combination thereof; cross-links of an inappropriate nature result in artery rigidity and skin wrinkling.

Cysteine—sulfur-containing amino acid.

Cystocele—hernia of the bladder, resulting in its protrusion into the vagina.

Diuretic—agent that promotes the excretion of urine.

Diverticulitis—inflammation of a part of the intestines, usually causing crampy pain in the lower left side of the abdomen.

DNA—abbreviation for deoxyribonucleic acid, the fundamental component of living matter.

Dopamine—important brain neurotransmitter that plays a role in body movement, motivation, primitive drives, sexual behavior, emotions, and immune system function.

Double-blind study—study in which neither the experimenter nor the subjects know who is getting what treatment.

Dysmenorrhea—painful or difficult menstruation.

Edema—excessive accumulation of fluid in tissues, causing swelling.

Endocrine glands—glands that manufacture hormones and release them into the bloodstream (such as adrenal glands, ovaries, and pancreas).

Endorphins—natural opiatelike substances in the brain that control pain, among other things.

Enzyme—protein capable of producing or accelerating a specific biochemical reaction at body temperature.

Epidemiological study—study of the occurrence and prevalence of disease.

Estrogen—class of female sex hormones found in both men and women, but in larger proportions in women; primarily responsible for the development and maintenance of female sex characteristics and reproductive functions in women.

Estrone—weaker form of estrogen.

Fibroids—fibrous, noncancerous growths most commonly found in or on the uterus.

Follicle—small, round sac; in the ovary, each egg is contained in a follicle.

Follicle-stimulating hormone (FSH)—hormone secreted by the pituitary gland that stimulates the follicles in the ovary to grow and mature.

Free radicals—highly reactive molecular fragments, generally harmful to the body.

Gamma-linolenic acid (GLA)—polyunsaturated fat that is used by the body to produce certain prostaglandins that control several important body processes.

Glucose—simple sugar that is the usual form in which the carbohydrate exists in the bloodstream.

Glucose tolerance factor (GTF)—a chromium compound that aids insulin in the control of blood sugar.

Glycogen—principal form in which a carbohydrate is stored in the body for ready conversion into energy; found in the liver and muscle tissue in particular.

Hemoglobin—protein in the blood that contains iron and carries oxygen from the lungs to the tissues.

Histamine—compound, found in many tissues, that is responsible for the increased permeability of blood vessels and plays a major role in allergic reactions.

Homeostasis—body's tendency to maintain a steady state of equilibrium despite external changes.

Hormone—chemical substance produced in one part of the body and carried in the blood to another part of the body, where it has specific effects.

Hydrogenation—addition of hydrogen to any unsaturated compound (oils are changed to solid fats by this process).

Hypoglycemia—low or falling concentration of glucose in the bloodstream, often caused by an excessive intake of refined carbohydrates in the diet.

Hypothalamus—part of the brain containing groups of nerve cells that control temperature, sleep, water balance, and other chemical and visceral activities.

Hysterectomy—surgical removal of the uterus (a radical hysterectomy includes removal of the uterus, cervix, ovaries, egg tubes, and sometimes lymph nodes near the ovaries).

Incontinence—inability to control urine retention.

Insulin—protein hormone secreted by the pancreas into the blood; regulates carbohydrate, fat, and protein metabolism.

Kyphosis—humpback or curvature of the spine in an anterior-posterior position.

Labia majora—major lips or folds of skin of the female external genitals, located on either side of the entrance to the vagina.

Lactase—intestinal enzyme that breaks down lactose (a sugar) into easily digested compounds.

Lactobacillus acidophilus—class of "friendly" bacteria found in yogurt and other milk products; also found in both the intestines and the vagina, where it controls the growth of yeast.

Lactose—sugar found in milk and other dairy products.

Lactose intolerance—deficiency of the lactase enzyme, which results in uncomfortable gastrointestinal symptoms when foods containing lactose are eaten.

Lecithin—waxlike substance with emulsifying and antioxidant properties, found distributed in animals and plants.

Libido—A Freudian term for the sexual drive or the energy of primitive biological urges.

Lordosis—inward curvature of the lower spine.

Luteinizing hormone (LH)—hormone produced by the pituitary (a large surge of this hormone in each menstrual cycle precedes ovulation by 12 to 24 hours).

Menarche—beginning of menstruation.

Metabolism—sum of chemical changes; the building up or destruction of cells that takes place in the body.

Neurotransmitter—substance that transmits nerve impulses across a synapse; brain chemicals that are involved in carrying messages to and from the brain.

Oophorectomy—removal of the ovaries (also called ovariectomy).

Ovary—one of two female organs containing the eggs and the cells that produce the female hormones estrogen and progesterone.

Ovulation—process during which a mature egg is released from the ovary.

Oxalates—compounds that can interfere with the absorption of calcium; found in some leafy green vegetables, such as spinach.

Oxidation—process of combining with oxygen.

Pancreas—large, glandular organ, extending across the upper abdomen close to the liver, that secretes digestive juices into the intestinal tract, which contains enzymes that act upon protein, fat, and carbohydrates; also secretes the hormone insulin directly into the blood.

Phytates—phosphorus-containing compounds that can interfere with the absorption of calcium; found in the outer husk of cereal grains.

Pituitary gland—small, oval organ, at the base of the brain that produces many important hormones (particularly FSH and LH) and has been called "the master gland."

Placebo—pill having no medicinal value, often used as a control in an experimental situation.

Polyps—soft, red growths with stems that most commonly occur in organs such as the uterus and rectum; usually noncancerous but can cause a discharge or can bleed when irritated.

Progesterone—hormone produced by the ovary during the second half of the menstrual cycle; promotes the growth of the uterine lining prior to menstruation and, in pregnancy, the growth of the placenta.

Progestogens—group of steroid hormones that include progesterone and other hormones that have similar effects.

Prolapse—the falling down (out of position) of an organ.

Prostaglandins—one of several compounds formed from essential fatty acids and whose activities affect the nervous, circulatory, and reproductive systems and metabolism. Research indicates that a type of prostaglandin is implicated in muscular contractions and menstrual cramps.

Rectocele—protrusion of the rectum into the vagina.

RNA (ribonucleic acid)—compound of nucleic acid responsible for the transmission of inherited traits.

Serotonin—substance present in many tissues (especially the blood and nerve tissue) that stimulates a variety of smooth muscles and nerves and is believed to function as a neurotransmitter.

Syndrome—set of symptoms that occur together.

Testosterone—strongest of the male sex hormones, found in both women and men, but in much greater proportions in men.

Thyroid gland—organ at the base of the neck primarily responsible for regulating the rate of metabolism.

Tryptophan—essential amino acid useful in treating sleep disorders and depression.

Tubal ligation—procedure that surgically blocks the fallopian tubes, preventing the union of sperm and egg.

Urethrocele—overgrowth of the fibrous tissue surrounding the urethra (the outlet from the bladder).

Uterus—complex female organ composed of smooth muscle and glandular lining; the womb.

Vagina—muscular canal in the female that extends from the vulva to the cervix.

Vasodilation—enlargement or dilation of blood vessels.

Vulva—external female sex organ, composed of the major and minor lips (labia majora and minora), the clitoris, and the opening of the vagina.

RESOURCES

———————— ❧ ————————

BEAUTY

Vera's Natural Beauty Retreat, Inc.
18670 Ventura Blvd.
Tarzana, CA 91356
Vera Brown, with Patricia Culligan, *Vera Brown's Natural Beauty Book* (Mountain View, CA: Anderson World Books, 1981).

Tovar's
9756 Wilshire Blvd.
Beverly Hills, CA 20210

BOOKLETS

Virginia Fontana et al., *Charting Your Way Thru PMS* (Claremont, CA: Hunter House Inc., Publishers, 1985)

Maria Lopez et al., *Menopause: A Self Care Manual* (Santa Fe, NM: A Santa Fe Health Education Project)

DIET

Benjamin T. Burton, *The Heinz Handbook of Nutrition* (New York: Mc-Graw-Hill, 1976).

Marin Katahn, Ph.D., *The 200 Calorie Solution* (New York: Berkley Books, 1982).
Susie Orbach, *Fat Is a Feminist Issue* (New York: Berkley Books, 1978).

Bobbe Sommer, Ph.D., *Not Another Diet Book* (Claremont, CA: Hunter House, 1986).

EXERCISE

Bob Anderson, *Stretching* (Bolinas, CA: Shelter Publications, 1980).

Sheila Cluff with Eve Shaw, *Sheila Cluff's Aerobic Body Contouring: The New Low-Impact Exercise Program for the Ageless Body* (Emmaus, PA, Rodale Press, 1987).

Covert Bailey, *Fit or Fat* (Boston: Houghton Mifflin, 1977).

Kenneth Cooper, M.D., *The New Aerobics* (New York: Bantam Books, 1970).

Jane Fonda with Mignon McCarthy, *Women Coming of Age* (New York: Simon & Schuster, 1984).

R. Hittleman, *Richard Hittleman's Yoga: 28-Day Exercise Plan*, New York: Bantam Books, 1969).

GENERAL INFORMATION AND INTEREST

Boston Women's Health Book Collective, *The New Our Bodies, Ourselves* (New York: Simon & Schuster, 1984).

Anne Morrow Lindbergh, *Gift from the Sea* (New York: Pantheon, 1955).

Kaylan Pickford, *Always A Woman* (New York: Bantam Books, 1982).

Andrew Weil, *Health and Healing* (Boston: Houghton Mifflin, 1983).

GYNECOLOGICAL PROBLEMS

Barbara Edelstein, M.D., *The Woman Doctor's Medical Guide for Women* (New York: William Morrow, 1982).

Federation of Feminist Women's Health Centers, *A New View of a Woman's Body* (New York: Simon & Schuster, 1981).

Niels Lauersen, M.D., and Eileen Stukane, *Listen to Your Body: A Gynecologist Answers Women's Most Intimate Questions* (New York: Berkley Books, 1982).

L. Madaras et al., *Womancare: A Gynecologic Guide to Your Body* (New York: Avon, 1981).

HEALTH RESORTS

The Oaks at Ojai
122 East Ojai Avenue
Ojai, CA 93023
(805) 646-5573

The Palms at Palm Springs
572 N. Indian Avenue
Palm Springs, CA 92262
(619) 325-1111

MENOPAUSE CLINICS

Center for Climacteric Studies
University of Florida
901 N.W. 8th Avenue, Suite B1
Gainesville, FL 32601

NEWSLETTERS

Hot Flash: Newsletter for Midlife and Older Women
Edited by Jane Porcino, Ph.D.
School of Allied Health Professionals
State University of New York
Stony Brook, NY 11794

Midlife Wellness
Center for Climacteric Studies
University of Florida
901 N.W. 8th Avenue, Suite B1
Gainesville, FL 32061

NUTRITION

Jeffrey Bland, *Nutraerobics: Dr. Jeffrey Bland's Complete Individualized Nutrition and Fitness Program for Life After 30* (San Francisco: Harper & Row, 1983).

Mark Bricklin, *The Natural Healing Cookbook* (Emmaus, PA: Rodale Press, 1981).

Patricia Housman, *The Right Dose: How to Take Vitamins and Minerals Safely* (Emmaus, PA: Rodale Press, 1987).

F. M. Lappe, *Diet for a Small Planet: Tenth Anniversary Edition* (New York: Ballantine Books, 1982).

L. Robertson et al., *Laurel's Kitchen: A Handbook for Vegetarian Cookery and Nutrition* (Petaluma, CA: Nilgiri Press, 1976).

PAMPHLETS

"Menopause" (Washington, DC: National Women's Health Network)

Robin Van Liew, "Herbal Remedies for Women" (New York: Feminist Health Works, 1980)

INDEX

ORDER FORM

NAME

ADDRESS

CITY   STATE

ZIP   COUNTRY

TITLE	QTY	PRICE	TOTAL
Charting Your Way	@	$3.95	
The Enabler	@	$6.95	
Exclusively Female	@	$5.95	
Healthy Aging *(paperback)*	@	$11.95	
Healthy Aging *(hard cover)*	@	$17.95	
Menopause Without Medicine	@	$11.95	
Not Another Diet Book	@	$15.95	
Nutrition and Your Body	@	$9.95	
Once A Month	@	$8.45	
Raising Each Other	@	$7.95	

Shipping costs:
*First book: $2.00
($3.00 for Canada)
Each additional
book: $.50 ($.75
for Canada)
For UPS rates and
bulk orders call us
at (714) 624-2277*

TOTAL	
Less discount @_____%	(_____)
TOTAL COST OF BOOKS	
Calif. residents add sales tax	
Shipping & handling	
TOTAL ENCLOSED *Please pay in U.S. funds only*	

❑ Check   ❑ Money Order   ❑ Visa   ❑ M/C

Card # _____ Exp date _____

Signature _____

Complete and mail to:

Hunter House Inc., Publishers

PO Box 847, Claremont, CA 91711

❑ Check here to receive our book catalog